Personal Computing for
Health Professionals

Personal Computing for Health Professionals

PHILIP BURNARD
University of Wales College of Medicine
Cardiff, UK

CHAPMAN & HALL
London · Glasgow · New York · Tokyo · Melbourne · Madras

Published by Chapman & Hall, 2-6 Boundary Row, London SE1 8HN

Chapman & Hall, 2-6 Boundary Row, London SE1 8HN, UK

Blackie Academic & Professional, Wester Cleddens Road, Bishopbriggs, Glasgow G64 2NZ, UK

Chapman & Hall Inc., 29 West 35th Street, New York NY10001, USA

Chapman & Hall Japan, Thomson Publishing Japan, Hirakawacho Nemoto Building, 6F, 1-7-11 Hirakawa-cho, Chiyoda-ku, Tokyo 102, Japan

Chapman & Hall Australia, Thomas Nelson Australia, 102 Dodds Street, South Melbourne, Victoria 3205, Australia

Chapman & Hall India, R. Seshadri, 32 Second Main Road, CIT East, Madras 600 035, India

Distributed in the USA and Canada by Singular Publishing Group Inc., 4284 41st Street, San Diego, California 92105

First edition 1993

© 1993 Philip Burnard

Typeset in 10.5/13pt Palatino by Excel Typesetters Company Ltd, Hong Kong
Printed in Great Britain by Clays Ltd, Bungay

ISBN 0 412 49670 4   1 56593 149 1 (USA)

Apart from any fair dealing for the purposes of research or private study, or criticism or review, as permitted under the UK Copyright Designs and Patents Act, 1988, this publication may not be reproduced, stored, or transmitted, in any form or by any means, without the prior permission in writing of the publishers, or in the case of reprographic reproduction only in accordance with the terms of the licences issued by the Copyright Licensing Agency in the UK, or in accordance with the terms of licences issued by the appropriate Reproduction Rights Organization outside the UK. Enquiries concerning reproduction outside the terms stated here should be sent to the publishers at the London address printed on this page.
  The publisher makes no representation, express or implied, with regard to the accuracy of the information contained in this book and cannot accept any legal responsibility or liability for any errors or omissions that may be made.

A catalogue record for this book is available from the British Library

∞ Printed on permanent acid-free text paper, manufactured in accordance with the proposed ANSI/NISO Z 39.48-199X and ANSI Z 39.48-1984

For my son, Aaron, for all his help

Contents

Acknowledgements	x
Introduction	**1**
A few words about words	1
Who is this book for?	2
Aims of the book	2
What is in the book?	3
How to use the book	4
1 Personal computers and the health professional	**7**
Types of computers	8
Uses of personal computers in the health professions	10
Caring and computing	11
Further reading	15
2 Types and aspects of personal computers	**17**
What is a personal computer?	17
PC components	17
Desktop computers	29
Laptop computers	30
The notebook	31
Palmtop computers	35
Modems	35
Other add-ons	37
CD-ROM	38
Printers	38
What sort of computer should you buy?	40
Further reading	40

3 Buying and using a personal computer — 43
Changing from a PCW — 43
Potential user checklist — 44
How to find the right dealer — 45
Buying through the post — 46
Renting and leasing — 48
Buying secondhand — 48
Consumables — 50
Starting out — 51
Further reading — 51

4 Operating systems and housekeeping with the personal computer — 53
Operating systems — 53
DOS — 54
Windows — 57
Windows or DOS? — 60
Desqview — 61
What is 'housekeeping'? — 63
Further reading — 75

5 Wordprocessing — 77
What is wordprocessing? — 77
Uses in health care settings — 78
Varieties of wordprocessor — 78
Checklist of wordprocessing functions — 79
Collective writing — 86
Setting up your wordprocessor — 91
Further reading — 93

6 Databases — 95
Database programs: essentials — 95
Choosing a database — 96
Using databases in the health care professions — 98
The Data Protection Act — 100
Other database programs — 107
Health care databases: data on a compact disk — 107
Further reading — 112

7 Other software for health care professionals — 113
Spreadsheets — 113
Graphics — 120
Desktop publishing — 125
Buying software — 128
Further reading — 130

8 Shareware — 133
Advantages — 133
History of shareware — 134
Examples of shareware programs — 136
Further reading — 137

9 Writing skills — 139
Writing with a computer — 139
General principles of good writing — 139
Paragraph layout — 145
Style — 146
Applying the principles to wordprocessing — 147
Tips for wordprocessing with Windows programs — 152
Writing papers, articles and reports — 155
Writing books, dissertations and larger projects — 156
Further reading — 161

10 Research and the personal computer — 163
Planning your research project — 163
Data collection — 164
Data analysis — 167
Writing the report — 174
Further reading — 175

References — 177
Appendix 1 Glossary of computer terms — 179
Appendix 2 Examples of commercial software — 193
Appendix 3 Shareware — 209
Bibliography — 233
Index — 235

Acknowledgements

I am indebted to my son, Aaron, to whom this book is dedicated. He has patiently taught me all about aspects of computing over the past few years and has put up with a good deal of my impatience. In a sense, this is as much his book as it is mine.

All trademarks are acknowledged, including those of computer software, books and any other publications. I am grateful to *PC Answers*, Future Publishing, Bath, for permission to reproduce the glossary that appears as an appendix in this book. Thanks to Premier Shareware, Orpington, Kent, for permission to reproduce material about the history of shareware in Chapter 8 and details of shareware programs in Appendix 3.

Acknowledgements are given to Dennis Publishing Ltd, London, for permission to reproduce details about commercial software in Appendix 2, from the June 1992 edition of *Computer Buyer*.

Introduction

All health professionals use computers at some point in their careers. Some like them and some loathe them. The aim of this book is to help to increase the former and decrease the latter. It is not a highly technical book but a practical one. From the user's point of view, a computer is a bit like a car. You don't need to know exactly how they work but you do need to know how to use and maintain them. This is a book about using and maintaining personal computers.

Personal computers – the stand-alone sort – can be useful in a wide range of applications in the health care field, both for work purposes and for home use. This book illustrates some of the ways in which health care workers can use computers to help them organize their work and to generally make their working and home lives more interesting. For computers can save a lot of time. They can also waste a lot if you have to spend hours trying to find out how aspects of them work. It is hoped that this book will get you started fairly quickly and will help you make decisions about the sort of computer you need and want.

A FEW WORDS ABOUT WORDS

Computing, like all other fields, has developed its own jargon. I have tried to keep the use of this jargon to a minimum. There are certain words, though, that are unavoidable. Let me clarify just two. **Hardware** refers to the equipment that makes up a computer system: the keyboard, the monitor, the chips and so on. **Software** refers to the programs that you run on a computer. Examples of software would be wordprocessing programs, like WordPerfect or Word for Windows.

These two words are so much a part of computing that you need to know about them straight away. Having said that, I have tried to avoid as many jargon words as possible in this book. It is not a technical manual, nor is it a guide to the darker recesses of your computer. It is a practical guide for people in the health professions who want to use computers. Or those who do not particularly want to do so, but have to!

WHO IS THIS BOOK FOR?

The book is for any health professional who needs or wants to use a computer. A short list of likely readers includes:

- students
- teachers, tutors and lecturers
- clinical workers
- nurses
- doctors
- social workers
- physiotherapists
- counsellors
- occupational therapists
- those in alternative therapies

This list is not meant to be exhaustive. The point is that the book will hopefully be useful to anyone who wants to use a computer but is not sure how to do so. It is also for those who do not want to wade through heavy manuals and computer magazines in order to find out how to get up and running. In the end, of course, everyone has to read the manuals at some point but that can usually come after an initial period of familiarization with the basic principles.

AIMS OF THE BOOK

This is an introductory text for a range of health care professionals. It aims to do the following:

- introduce you to a range of aspects of personal computing;
- offer you advice on how to select and buy a personal computer;
- help you to organize your hard disk;
- enable you to make decisions about what software you may want to buy from a range of commercially available programs and shareware;
- explain how to use wordprocessors, databases, spreadsheets and a range of other programs in a health care context;
- identify some of the ways that you can use a computer for writing essays, projects, books and larger reports;
- discuss some of the ways that you can use a personal computer to organize, analyse and report your research projects;
- help you to select other books to take your computing studies further.

WHAT IS IN THE BOOK?

The book focuses only on the personal computer. It does not cover mainframes or other varieties such as the Apple Macintosh, the Atari or the Amstrad PCW. This is not meant to imply that any of these computers is less useful than the PC, it is because the PC has become widely used in the health care professions and as a home and business computer.

Chapter 1 defines the personal computer and discusses its role in the health care professions. Chapter 2 takes a closer look at different options that are available, from desktops to notebooks, and helps you to make decisions about what you need to buy. Chapter 3 is about buying a computer, whilst Chapter 4 discusses 'housekeeping' – the process of managing your machine. The next three chapters are about different sorts of computer program and how they might best be used. Chapter 8 introduces shareware – a unique marketing strategy in the business world which allows you to try programs before you buy them. The final two chapters offer practical advice about using a personal computer for writing and doing research.

There are boxes throughout the book, called Computing Tips, which identify things to consider when using your computer. There are examples and descriptions of programs and other software that may be useful, at various points in the book. These are included to offer concrete examples of the principles under discussion. All the programs that I have described are ones I have used myself in my job as a health care lecturer and as a writer. Clearly, others are also available and lists of software and shareware are included in the appendices.

As noted above, the point of the book is that it should be practical. It does not cover all aspects of computing (networks and modems, for example, are not discussed in depth). Instead, I have tried to identify those issues that will be of immediate value to any health care professional who needs to learn to use a computer fairly quickly. Whilst it can never replace hands-on experience of sitting at a keyboard, I hope that it will be useful as a companion. I would emphasize that the book is not intended to replace computer or software manuals, nor is it meant to be an authoritative guide to the inner workings of a computer. I am a university lecturer with a particular interest in communication and I have written the book with this focus in mind. The point of computers, for me, is that they can enhance communication in almost all spheres of the health care field.

HOW TO USE THE BOOK

If you want, you can read the book through at one sitting. Whilst this is obviously recommended with novels, it is rarely the best way to use non-fiction books. Probably the most useful way of approaching this book, if you have not used a computer so far, is to read the first two chapters and then pick out the other chapters that you need, as you need them. If you are familiar with the basics of computing, you may want to skip read the early chapters and move straight to those about practical applications. Hopefully, too, the book is one that you can use as a reference to return to when you need to upgrade or change your computer.

At the time of writing, the computer world is in a state of flux. New processors and new machines are coming onto the market every week. Prices are still dropping. For this reason, I have avoided reference to particular processors and particular machines, except in passing. I have not made any reference to prices as this sort of information is likely to be irrelevant by the time you pick up the book. The book, then, is about practical principles and not about pricing or technical details. Also, it is a personal view. The methods I describe in this book are ones that I have found useful but they are never the only way of doing things.

One of the most exciting and yet ironic aspects of computing is this: that whatever you read in a book about computing is likely to be wrong. This is simply because the field is still changing so rapidly. Alongside the reading of this book, you will have to constantly check the current state of things as they are at this moment. All computer books necessarily become historical documents very quickly. That need not, I hope, stop them from being useful.

Writing for the person who is completely new to computing is difficult. Inevitably, special words or jargon creep in. As far as possible, I have tried to explain all of this jargon as it occurs in the text. If, however, you spot words that you do not know, look in the glossary at the back of the book and this will offer you a definition of the particular word.

Computing can become compulsive. Whilst no one would wish a compulsion on you, I hope that you find the book useful and that you enjoy using computers.

Philip Burnard
Caerphilly
Mid Glamorgan

Personal computers and the health professional

Computers are now central instruments in the health care field and they can be enjoyable to use. To some, computers seem out of place in the health care professions. They spell 'technology' in a rather unpleasant way. They appear to be invading the personal and professional relationship between client and helper. Another way of viewing them, however, is as useful tools that free you to devote more time to what you really have to do. Rather than get in the way of relationships, their ability to do quickly what humans do slowly can be a major advantage. Consider, for example, the following situations in which computers can help immediately:

- Wordprocessing: if you have to write papers, essays or simply notes, wordprocessing can mean never having to rewrite from scratch.
- Databases: if you need to keep and change records of any sort, a computer will often be the quickest and most economical way of doing this.
- Spreadsheets: if you have to keep accounts, a spreadsheet can take most of the arithmetic out of your accounts keeping.
- Graphics packages: if you have to illustrate a research report with bar or pie charts, a graphics package can help you make these look professional.
- Statistics packages: statistics can be calculated very quickly with the use of a computer statistics program. The package will never make you a statistician, but it will do the calculation for you, if you know the criteria for running the tests.

Some people are still frightened of computers. Some feel that they have missed the technological revolution and are too old to begin to learn about them. Just by way of an aside, I hadn't touched a computer until I was 30 and was sure that I would never be able to use one. Once I began to learn, I realized that I was unlikely to return to a pad and pen as a major method of writing. Yet other people worry about breaking their computers. If you drop them, you are likely to; just pressing the wrong keys almost never has a lasting effect. Almost all of the errors you make at the keyboard can be rectified easily. There are relatively few moving parts in a computer so the possibility of damage is extremely limited. Also, and rather surprisingly, parts for computers are fairly cheap. Keyboards, for example, cost little more than computer books. If you do spill coffee all over one, you can fairly easily replace it.

The keyword, throughout the process of learning about computers, should be **experience**. You cannot learn computing from a book: you need hands-on experience. This book makes no attempt to replace the manuals that come with your computer nor those that come with your programs. Its aim, instead, is to show you some of the ways in which you can make computers a more central part of your personal and professional life. My contention is that they can free you to offer more time to your clients, your colleagues and your family. If, that is, you don't become so hooked on them that you end up spending more time with them than you do with all of these people. For computers can also be seductive; there have already been articles about 'computer widows'. The point is to use them wisely and to use them for work. The only real danger is in becoming a 'computer tinkerer' – a person who fiddles with all of the minor details of a program or with the setting up of the machine to the degree that little productive work gets done. Learn what you need to about computers. In the first place, learn enough to get you started. Then, as your needs increase, explore the computing world more fully.

TYPES OF COMPUTERS

Anyone who wants to buy a computer is faced with a considerable series of choices. First, what sort of computer do you want? Note that not all types of computers are compatible with each other. For example, it is possible to buy the following types of computer that all run in rather different ways:

- the IBM and compatible personal computer
- the Apple Macintosh
- the Atari
- the Amstrad wordprocessor
- the Archimedes

Whilst it is usually possible to buy 'add-ons' that make it possible for each of these computers to read one another's disks, this is not automatically possible. You can't take a disk out of an Amstrad wordprocessor, slot it straight into an Apple Macintosh and expect to be able to read what is on the disk. For that reason, and because they are used so widely, this book is **only** about IBM, and compatible, personal computers. That is not to say that they are an improvement on the others, necessarily easier to use or more efficient. You are advised to explore the whole range of computers if you can and thus to make an informed choice about which one you buy. If you are to use one at work, of course, the decision may be made for you: the hospital or organization in which you are working is likely to make the decision to install only one sort of computer throughout all of the departments. They may also decide to set up a **network** system – the means of linking computers together so that department can talk to department and data can be shared. If this happens, then it seems reasonable to buy a similar sort of computer for home use. To use one sort of machine at work and another at home means that you have two sets of commands to learn: you have to know how to 'work' both sorts of computers. Make life a bit easy: settle for one sort of computer. Many health authorities make the decision to install either IBM compatible machines or Apple Macintoshes. The other sorts of computers, mentioned above, are more often used as 'stand-alone' machines, either for the home market or for business use. The Amstrad wordprocessor has been adopted for use by a lot of home computer buyers but it looks as though its life will be limited. It incorporates old technology and the price of IBM compatible machines is dropping so dramatically that the Amstrad wordprocessor is no longer the bargain it was in 1987.

USES OF PERSONAL COMPUTERS IN THE HEALTH PROFESSIONS

What can you use a personal computer for? Here is a shortlist of possible uses in the health professions:

- letter writing
- storage of patient/client records
- preparation of lecture notes
- storage of bibliographical references
- paper, article and book writing
- project preparation
- keeping of accounts
- preparation of graphics presentations
- preparation of conferences notes
- development of curriculum packages
- preparation of handouts and book lists
- production of newsletters
- preparation of small posters and fly sheets
- automation of prescription writing
- doing statistics in research
- editing other people's written work.

Most of the things that can be done with a pen and paper can be done better with a computer. Pfaffenberger (1991) suggests that the automation offered by a personal computer can be viewed as the means by which skills formerly possessed only by highly paid experts are made available to many people. He sums up an example of this 'redistribution of skills' like this:

> Word processing software is an excellent example of the potential of automation to distribute skills; a secretary can expertly centre text on the page and proofread spelling so that letters and reports contain no spelling or typographical errors. A high-quality word processing program such as WordPerfect is, in part, an automated secretary,

and its economic significance lies partly in the fact that the program brings secretarial expertise to people and small businesses that could not afford such expertise in the past.

I hope that this book illustrates some of the ways in which this sharing of expertise can permeate the health care professions via the personal computer.

Computing Tip 1

Make regular back-ups

You must back up the data on your hard disk to floppy disk for storage. If the hard disk fails, if you do not have a copy of your work, you may have no data. Many people assume that hard disks run for ever. They do not and at some point they 'crash'. Make sure that everything that you have on your hard disk could also be found on floppies. There is usually no need to back up all the programs on your hard disk as you will already have the original disks.

This issue is so fundamental to computing, it is worth saying again, more strongly:

ALWAYS MAKE BACK-UPS!

The voice of doom: one day, you won't and you will regret it!

CARING AND COMPUTING

In some areas, there seems to be a reaction against technology in the health care professions. This may be seen in the flourishing of alternative therapies and in the encouragement of more 'intuitive' approaches to care. Part of this change has also been brought about by more and more health care professions questioning the 'medical model' as the only way of thinking about and working with health and illness. Indeed, we are seeing an increased interest in the notion of health as a central focus rather than illness. With that development has arisen 'new disciplines' such as health psychology. This period of change and upheaval runs parallel to considerable changes in the provision of health care. The past ten or so years have seen a revolution in the way health care provision is planned and delivered. Some have welcomed that revolution and others have been sceptical.

Also, there have been considerable changes in the training and education of health care professionals. There has been a move away from traditional 'information giving' teaching methods towards more student centred and experiential modes of learning. The accent, increasingly, has been on learning rather than on teaching. At last, it would seem, the message is getting through that the focus of the educational process should be the student rather than the teacher or even the information that is transmitted. Interestingly, it is in this field that computing can help considerably. Given that computers can store huge amounts of information that can be retrieved very quickly, the 'telling' part of education may well be delegated, at least to a small degree, to the computer. Meanwhile, health care educators and trainers can focus on the more 'human' and interactive aspects of their jobs. The value of computers in education is immediately recognizable in at least one field: the retrieval of bibliographic information in libraries. It is not unfair to say that the use of CD-ROM library facilities has revolutionized the ways in which literature searches can be carried out by students in any of the health care professions.

Meanwhile, in an entirely different domain, the computing world itself has also changed radically. As we have seen, miniaturization and the drop in cost of components has meant that more and more people have had access to computers. Nowadays, it is not at all unusual for people to have computers in their homes – not just for use as games machines but as aids to writing and business. We have also witnessed the development of new ways of working via the 'home-office'. Working at or from home is seen by some as a phenomenon which will become increasingly central for many of the people who remain in full and part time employment.

All this would appear to leave health care workers and people who work with computers at opposite ends of the spectrum. After all, if the health care professions are becoming more concerned with personal relationships, with health and with 'hands on' care, and if people who work with computers might be working from home and not directly alongside others, the two groups would seem to have little in common. I think, however, that a synthesis is possible. One of the most important features of the personal computer is its speed of operation. It is also relatively simple to operate. Its 'high tech' features are becoming easier to operate and easier to live with. We are becoming more and more familiar with computers and with what they can do. Nor do we have to know how they work. The analogy of a car is a simple but appropriate one. I know how to drive but I don't know much about the details of the engine in my car. I neither want nor need to know. So it is with computing. We do not need to know the details of chips and processors. We need to know how to make computers work for us. If we know that and are not frightened or dismissive of them, we can use them to free time for more of the things that we want to do in health care. The technology can enable us to spend more time on the more abstract but human and 'difficult' aspects of care: qualitative research, interpersonal relationships, discovering ways of encouraging positive health and so on.

Personal computers are becoming familiar objects in the health care field. They can be used in GP surgeries to free the GP by automating many of the routine administrative tasks, improve patient satisfaction by enhancing the service and can even help to problem solve in the question of diagnosis. In various hospitals and clinics, they are being used as the means of storing patient records and of planning care. Nursing Informatics is a growing field that covers all aspects of data handling but is particularly concerned with the use of personal computers in the delivery of skilled nursing care. In the future, the time saving and convenience features of the personal computer are likely to make it a necessary part of the health care scene.

Consider one example from my own field of teaching health care in a university setting. Anyone in a job like mine is expected to teach, to do research, to publish and to carry out some administrative duties. Consider, now, how a computer can make a difference to the ways in which some of those duties are carried out. Before having a personal computer to work on, I handwrote lecture notes and had them typed and photocopied, booked time on a mainframe computer to analyse data and wrote papers on blocks of A4 feint and margin which were later typed out (and, if necessary, retyped) by a secretary as a 'low priority' task. I wrote my first book on a series of A4 pads and that too was typed, part time, by a secretary. The whole process of producing a manuscript suitable for sending to a publisher took a couple of years. Nowadays, I not only write direct to the screen but I can also send a manuscript to a publisher on disk. The same is true of journal papers. Many journals and professional magazines will accept manuscripts on disk and at least one encourages the sending of manuscripts via a modem – from the computer to the publisher down the telephone line.

Finally, the question of administration. I run a variety of Masters degree courses. The administration of these takes up a considerable amount of time. However, I can now delegate some of that time to the computer through the use of student databases, standard letters, edited reading lists and other course materials. All of this means that I can spend more time in the areas that need time: teaching and 'hands-on' research. In this latter activity, the fact of having a personal computer always to hand makes a considerable difference. In a recent study about AIDS counselling that I undertook (Burnard, 1992), I was able to transcribe interviews directly onto a laptop computer, thus bypassing the recording and more traditional forms of interview transcription. I had organized the computer software before I undertook the interviews in such a way as to make content analysis of those interviews a relatively straightforward process. The final write-up of subsequent papers and a book was all carried out on the same computer. The manuscript of the book was delivered to the publisher as 'camera ready copy'. Again, a saving of time and a short-circuiting of some of the more traditional processes of publication.

The picture is not a completely rosy one. Learning to use computers takes up time. It is important to use them efficiently and to learn how to make best use of them. It is not a good idea to use them as glorified typewriters, for this is to waste their potential. Also, they need to be looked after. Data on hard disks needs to be backed up regularly; 'housekeeping' tasks (such as the ones described in this book) must be carried out. Computers can also go wrong. When they do, they can go wrong in spectacular ways. I recently spent an anxiety ridden afternoon rescuing data 'blind' from a hard disk when an important connection between the computer and the monitor became faulty. This meant that I couldn't see anything on the screen and had to 'feel' my way around the hard disk, via the keyboard. It was all a very hit and miss affair but I managed to rescue important files, transfer them to floppies and work on them on another machine. I don't like to think what might have happened if I could not have retrieved them.

All in all, though, the benefits of working with computers far outweigh any problems they may present. They do not have to be the domain of a few knowledgeable 'techies'. I am convinced that almost anyone can learn to use them and that they have a positive contribution to make to health care work. Their sheer ability to store and make accessible large amounts of information must contribute a considerable amount to the caring process. They should be seen as allies in the care of other people.

Computing Tip 2	**Use wide margins when writing with your wordprocessor** If you set the margins on your wordprocessor wide, you will be able to scan what you have written far more quickly. Also, some wordprocessors make the text disappear off the edge of the screen, by default. Consider using margin settings of 2" right and left whilst you are editing your work. When you want to print out, readjust your margins to the more normal 1" settings.

FURTHER READING

Pfaffenberger, B. (1991) *Que's Computer User's Dictionary*, Que Corporation, distributed by Computer Manuals Ltd, 50 James Road, Tyseley, Birmingham B11 2BA

Anyone who uses computers soon discovers that the computing world has a jargon all of its own. There are any number of computing dictionaries which will tell you what the jargon words really mean. This one is different in that it tells you in words that you can understand. It also offers much more than that.

Computer User's Dictionary is just that; a dictionary for users. It doesn't just define words, it also offers you a considerable amount of advice about how to use what you have just read. It is full of tips on how to get the best performance out of your computer and, in this respect, it is more like an encyclopaedia than a dictionary. The entries in it, for many words and phrases, are much longer than the ones you find in most dictionaries. This is because of the amount of information that it offers. And it is soon apparent that the author is a real authority. You quickly get to feel that you can depend on the advice that you are being given. Once you start putting that advice into practice, you see that he really is an authority.

This book should be on the bookshelf of anyone who uses computers. Because it offers you advice as well as definitions, it is the sort of book that you can turn to in crises and when programs are not running to order. It is much more than a dictionary; it is a lifeline.

2 Types and aspects of personal computers

There are a number of decisions to be made by anyone considering buying a computer. This chapter discusses some of the parts that go to make up a computer and some of the types of personal computers that are available. It also contains various checklists that will help you to make your mind up about what sort of computer you need.

WHAT IS A PERSONAL COMPUTER?

A personal computer is a stand-alone computer that is equipped with all the basic software to enable it to function and all the input and output devices that enable it to perform various computing tasks. The term 'personal computer' is normally reserved for those that developed out of the original IBM machine introduced in the early 1980s. Synonyms include 'IBM compatible', 'IBM clone' or simply 'PC'. The personal computer can be contrasted with other computers such as those made by Atari, Archimedes and Apple Macintosh. They are also different from the dedicated wordprocessing home computer made by Amstrad.

A point needs to be made at the outset, which will be taken up in more detail later: you can't simply buy a computer, switch it on and begin to type into it. A computer needs certain software to make it run – a disk operating system (DOS). It then needs specific software to enable the computer to do the task you want (a wordprocessing program or a spreadsheet program, for example).

PC COMPONENTS

There are three main components to a personal computer: the central processing unit (or box that contains the chips and drives), the keyboard and the monitor. There are decisions that need to be made about each of these and they are now discussed.

Central processing unit (CPU)

Strictly speaking, the term 'central processing unit' refers to the main microprocessing chip that is at the heart of the computer. Increasingly, it has come to refer to the box that contains all the chips, drives and memory. Usually, that box is separate from the monitor and sits underneath it. Sometimes, the unit is placed underneath a desk or table and sometimes it is stood on its end to make more room. If you intend to place yours in this position, you should check with the manufacturer that the computer can run in this way. Some hard disks are not made to run in a vertical plane and care should be taken in setting up your computer in this position. If you are a purist, and don't like the phrase 'central processing unit' used in this way, refer to it simply as 'the box'.

The processor

The processor is the chip at the centre of your computer. It is the real 'central processing unit' and has been described as the 'computer on a chip'. It has the single biggest influence on the performance of your machine. Computers in the early 1980s contained 8086 processors which drove computers called XTs. These were replaced by faster chips, known as 80286s, which were at the heart of ATs. The late 1980s saw the introduction of the 80386 family of chips and then the 80486s. The speed rating of a microprocessor chip is measured in megahertz (MHz) or millions of cycles per second. The original IBM PC in the early 1980s ran at 4.7MHz, whilst some 80486s run at 50MHz. In between those extremes are a range of processors that run at between 20 and 30MHz. The situation is changing by the month and at the time of writing, there appears to be no slowing down in the development of faster chips. Therefore, no attempt is being made here to recommend a particular chip or a particular computer. For most people, a faster machine will be preferable to a slower one. It will also cost more. Microprocessor speed also needs to be considered in relation to what you will use the computer for. If you are only going to use a DOS-based wordprocessor[1], then the

---

[1] See Chapter 4 for an explanation of DOS and Chapter 5 for a discussion about word-processing.

extra speed of an up-to-the-minute machine may not be used to the full. On the other hand, if you intend to do intensive work with graphics or with spreadsheet and database programs, the extra speed will be noticeable. Also, you need to make sure that if you buy a fast processor, the computer also comes with a fast hard disk. Like most machines, computers are let down by the weakest component in the chain. A computer that has a very fast microprocessor and a slow hard disk will not work as quickly as one with a fairly fast processor and a fast hard disk.

Computing Tip 3

Buy computer magazines

Read computer magazines, on sale in any High Street newsagents. They are the easiest way of keeping track of what is a continually changing field. Most particularly, they reflect changes in the pricing of computing equipment and software. Examples of some of the magazines that are available include:

- *Windows*
- *PC Plus*
- *PC Answers*
- *PC Direct*
- *What Personal Computer?*
- *PC Magazine*
- *Computer Buyer*

Memory

Programs and current data (whilst the computer is switched on) all have to be 'housed' somewhere. They run in memory (RAM or random access memory). In the early days of PCs, the standard amount of memory which a computer had was 640 kilobytes (k). In the early 1980s, it was thought that this was likely to be all the memory that anyone would ever need. As a result, the DOS operating system, which allows programs to run (see below), can only address 640k of memory unless you use a memory management program. A particularly powerful and useful one is QEMM by Quarterdeck. On the other hand, most PCs now come with at least 1 megabyte (Mb) and many are supplied with 4Mb as standard. The same principle applies: you can only use the first 640k unless you install a memory management program which allows your computer to address the memory above that.

Someone once said that you can never be too rich or too thin. In the computing world, you can never have too much memory. Extra memory (and the accompanying management system) can speed up your computing. The more memory you have, the less the computer has to refer to your hard or floppy disks for information. Also, with larger amounts of RAM, you can store what are known as 'terminate and stay resident' (TSR) programs. These are small programs that sit in memory and can be called up 'over' your current program by pressing a couple of keys. Your 'current' program stays exactly as it was when you left it: the TSR program simply pops up over it. There are a variety of TSR programs including notebooks, simple database programs, dictionaries and books of quotations. If, for example, you are writing a paper in your database, you can call up your dictionary program over the top of your word-processing program, check a spelling or a definition and return to the point that you left you paper. Examples of TSR programs include Sidekick by Borland and Oxford Writer's Shelf by Oxford University Press.

Random Access Memory (RAM), in a computer with more than 1Mb of memory, is composed of two areas: conventional memory (memory up to 1Mb) and extended memory (memory above 1Mb). However, the DOS operating system can normally only recognize the first 640k of conventional memory. To handle memory above that point, you need a memory manager such as QEMM by Quarterdeck. This program first allows you to use the memory between 640k and 1Mb to run certain parts of your operating system, hard disk drives and so on. This area, just above the 640k mark, is called high memory. A memory manager also allows you to access extended memory – memory above 1Mb. This can be used by a variety of programs, some of which can only use that extra memory if it is converted into expanded memory. A program such as QEMM works dynamically and enables memory above 1Mb to be configured either as extended or expanded memory according to particular programs' needs. Figure 2.1 illustrates the relationship between these different types of memory. Fortunately, for most of the time, you don't have to worry about the ins and outs of different types of memory: a

PC components

Extended Memory (can be transformed into Expanded Memory)	Above 1 Mb
High Memory	641 k – 1024 k (1 Mb)
Conventional Memory	0 – 640 k

Figure 2.1 Different types of memory.

program like QEMM sorts all of your memory problems out for you, automatically. Suffice it to say here that if you find that you need extra memory, it can usually be added to your computer in the form of plug-in chips.

Example software: **Sidekick 11 (Borland)**

Sidekick is a computer organizer. It is rather like having a diary, a notepad and a range of other home and office utilities to hand, at any given moment. It offers a whole range of features that anyone with a computer is likely to find useful.

First, the notepad feature. This is a mini wordprocessor that is easily as powerful as some other stand-alone wordprocessors. It includes full printing facilities, cut and paste features and even a spell checker and thesaurus. It will also sort words or phrases alphabetically, 'backwards or forwards'. For some odd reason a word counter is not included. You can open up to nine documents at any given time and quickly move between them. You may want to use this if you are working on various drafts of a document or if you are working with notes. Each open notepad can hold about eight to ten pages of text.

The notepad is probably Sidekick's single most useful feature. It is useful for jotting down notes and reminders. It is also handy for printing out addresses and quick notes to the milkman. It can also be used in place of those little yellow stickers that tend to take over the wall. Instead of stickers, you write yourself notes in the notepad. These can then be saved to disk and recalled whenever you need them. The notes, once transferred to files, can also be read into other wordprocessors.

The program also gives you a useful name and address database. You can even dial up numbers from within the database if you have the right equipment. The program also works with a modem and will help you to communicate with other computer users who have modems.

Sidekick has a range of calculators: a general calculator, a business one and a scientific one. Together, these offer all the calculating power that anyone is likely to need outside a full blown statistics package. Having an ordinary calculator to hand at the computer is often useful. The fact that you don't have to close down your program to use it makes the Sidekick general calculator particularly valuable. In effect, it turns the numerical keypad on the keyboard into a 'real' calculator.

Sidekick is likely to appeal to computer users who like to keep everything on their computer. Clearly, the notepad feature is useful for jotting down notes in the middle of a computing session. I have some reservations about using the diary feature; most of us like to carry our diaries around with us. Unless you carry a notebook or palmtop computer with you at all times, the diary feature of Sidekick is likely to be less useful. For many, though, the notepad feature alone will more than justify buying this program.

Hard disk drives

Programs and data files have to be stored somewhere. Although they can be stored on floppy disks (see below) they are better stored inside the computer on a hard disk. A hard disk is a form of built-in data storage. The standard size for the average hard disk at the time of writing is 40Mb. Hard disks are available from 20Mb to many thousands of megabytes. A safe rule of thumb is to buy the biggest hard disk you can find. It is usual to find yourself filling even a large hard disk over a period of time.

Hard disks are one of the most fragile aspects of the computer. Any data that you have on them must be backed up on floppy disks. You do not have to copy all of the program files that are on your hard disk: you will have copies of the programs on the original floppies. You must back up any new files that you write and any that you make amendments to. It is dangerous to get complacent. It is tempting to think that hard disks, like most of the other components of a computer, 'go on for ever'. They

PC components

do not: hard disks eventually fail. The leading question is this: could you, at any time, reproduce all of the data that is currently on your hard disk? If you could not, then you need to do some backing up. There are a number of programs available that help you in the process of backing up. Such programs are usually able to make 'incremental' back-ups which means that they will search the hard disk for new data and only copy to floppies new files or files that have been modified. This sort of incremental backing up can save you a lot of time.

The hard disk contains the 'root' directory and all of the subdirectories that are described in Chapter 4. Hard disks are so much bigger than floppies that you cannot simply empty all your programs and your data files onto them. Those programs and files need to be organized. As we shall see, the way to do this is to create subdirectories: labelled subsections of the disk that help you to find your way around it. You may, for example, have separate subdirectories for your wordprocessing program, your database program and your data files. These may be called WORDPR, DATAB and DATA so that they are clearly recognizable. Some programs, when you install them on your hard disk, create their own subdirectories automatically during the process of installation.

If you find that you are filling up your hard disk, it is often possible to replace it with one that has a larger capacity. Alternatively, you may want to install a 'hardcard'. This is a hard disk built into a card that slips into one of the expansion slots inside your computer. This gives you immediate access to another 20, 40 or more megabytes of storage space. The best way, though, is to buy the right sized hard disk in the first place. Those who use Windows programs are likely to need larger hard disks than those who stay with DOS. Windows programs often take up considerable space on a hard disk and it is quite easy to fill a smaller hard disk with programs – leaving no space for your own data files. Think big. Also, think fast. Hard disks vary in the speed with which they can be accessed and with which they can find data and bring it into memory. A fast computer can be spoilt by a slow hard disk. Get the friend that you take with you to buy a hard disk to ask about the speed of the hard disk.

Example software: **Super Stor (Adstore)**

Most personal computer users will use or be contemplating buying a hard disk. A hard disk is one which holds anywhere between 20Mb and about 3000Mb of data and files. The advantages of such a disk are clear. First, you can store much more data on a hard disk than you can on floppies. Second, hard disks usually run much faster than floppies. Third, they allow you to keep all of your programs and a lot of your data on the computer at any given time. If you use a notebook or laptop computer, this means that you can take with you your wordprocessor, database and any other programs that you regularly use.

The problem is, hard disks fill up. Most people who start out with a 20Mb or 40Mb disk think that they will never fill it up. All that space! After using a 'floppies only' machine, such storage capacity seems vast. But modern programs eat up megabytes. In no time at all, you find you are searching the hard disk for files to take off – to allow you to free up extra space.

This is where Super Stor comes in. At a stroke, it allows you to almost double the size of your hard disk. It works by 'compressing' the files on your disk, automatically. Thus, a 20Mb hard disk becomes almost the equivalent of a 40Mb one. Also, all this compression seems to make little difference to the running speed of your computer. You can compress your programs as well as your files.

All this is particularly valuable if you are working on a computer that cannot easily be upgraded. Whilst many will allow you to fit a second hard disk, some will not. Typically, notebook computers only have room for one hard disk. In these cases, Super Stor is just what you need. You first load all your programs and the data files that go with them and then you simply sit back while Super Stor gives them a squeeze. Super Stor then works away, invisibly, in the background, holding your work in a compressed format and allowing you to work with it in a 'normal' format when you need to.

Some computer companies are now offering Super Stor already installed on their hard disks. This is both a good and a bad thing. On the one hand, it allows you to store twice as much data on a hard disk. On the other hand, it can let some manufacturers appear to be offering larger hard disks than they really are.

Floppy disk drives

Floppy disks are the ones that you put in and take out of your computer. Programs, when you buy them, come on floppy disks and you back up your data files to floppies. The standard size floppy disk is now 3½". The 3½" floppy disk comes in three main capacities: 720k, 1.44Mb and, more recently, 2.8Mb. Most of them, these days, are of the 1.44Mb variety (these are known as 'high density' disks). You may also find computers that take 5¼" disks. These, paradoxically, cannot contain so much data and hold either 380k or 1.2Mb. The larger disks are far less robust. The 3½" disks are contained in a tough plastic cover, whilst the larger ones really are 'floppy'.

Floppy disks come with built-in protection against overwriting. The smaller ones have a small plastic notch which you move until you can see light shining through the hole that is left. Once the notch is moved in this way, you cannot write new data to the disk but you can still copy data from it. On the larger disks, you have to stick a piece of tape over a small chunk that is cut into the side of the disk cover in order to write-protect it. It is worth write-protecting all of your program disks so that you cannot accidentally overwrite the files that run your wordprocessor, database or spreadsheet.

If you have a choice, it is still worth considering buying a computer that has both 5¼" and 3½" disk drives. This will mean that you can use either sized disks and may be useful if you are sent data on a disk or buy programs that are only supplied on one particular size of disk. Many companies supply their programs on both sized disks as a matter of course.

What do you use floppy disks for, if you have a hard disk? These are the main uses of the floppy disk:

- to carry data from one place to another;
- to hold program files – computer programs are supplied on floppy disks but most need to be transferred to a hard disk to work properly; some programs cannot work at all without a hard disk;
- to back up the contents of your hard disk.

In some ways, floppy disks need more care than hard disks, if only because they are transportable. Bray (1992) suggests the following tips for ensuring a long life for floppy disks:

- Protect them from extremes of heat and humidity, especially direct sunlight.

- Keep them in a clean environment and replace the jackets on 5¼" disks directly after use.
- Don't touch the disk surface or try to clean it.
- Don't bend or fold 5¼" disks or put paperclips on them.
- Don't put heavy objects on top of disks.
- Don't write on them or use an eraser on or near them.
- Protect them from magnetic fields. Airport security equipment is generally safe but manufacturers recommend you don't put disks through them.
- Clean the heads of your disk drive regularly.
- If your use floppy disks for back-up, test the back-up now and then to make sure it is really working.

The box

The box that contains all the parts of a desktop computer usually comes in one of two types: the desktop itself and the 'tower' variety. A desktop box often sits straight underneath the monitor or on a shelf. The tower box can sit on the floor next to the computer table. Do not assume, automatically, that you can simply turn a desktop computer box on its side and run it. Some hard disk drives are made to run in one or other of the types of boxes and do not take kindly to suddenly having to run in a different plane.

Some computer boxes are full size whilst others are slimline. The full size ones are usually the ones to buy if you know that you are likely to upgrade parts of your system. A larger box means more space inside and more 'expansion slots' – slots in which you can put things like modems, extra disk drives and, sometimes, memory. A slimline box is likely to have many of its components crammed into a fairly small space. These boxes can make the relatively simple task of adding more memory difficult. In a slimline box, you are likely to need very thin fingers to work around the wires and components.

Keyboard

The standard layout for a personal computer nowadays includes 102 keys. Normally, the 'typewriter' keys are to the left and 12 'function' keys are above them. The function keys are used in various programs to

PC components

> **Computing Tip 4**
>
> **Re-use computer disks that you don't use**
>
> Many computer magazines magazines have a free disk full of programs stuck to the front cover. If you find that you do not need to use these programs, reformat the disk, relabel it and use it as a back-up disk for your data.

invoke certain actions in those programs. Almost universally, pressing F1 produces a help menu which gives you further information about the program. Many programs supply cardboard overlays which fit above the function keys to indicate their use in that particular program. If you use one program a lot, it is worth sticking the carboard template to the keyboard so that it is always to hand. To the right of the typewriter keyboard is a set of cursor keys which allows you to move the cursor around the screen (the cursor is the 'light blob' on the screen that tells you 'where you are' in a document or program). On the far right is a set of numerical keys which double-up those on the top of the 'typewriter' section. At first glance, this set of numerical keys appears to offer a calculator function. When I first saw a PC keyboard, I imagined that those keys naturally gave you all the functions of a calculator. Not so. You have to buy a program that allows these keys to work in that way, otherwise, they simply type numbers on the screen. However, the layout of the number keys in this way helps in the entry of numerical data. Anyone who is familiar with using a calculator or even a modern cash register will find the layout helpful.

The keyboard is the most 'subjective' part of the computing set-up. Keyboards vary considerably in the amount of 'give' in the keys and even in the amount of noise that is generated when the keys are pressed. Some computers even have an electronic 'bleep' that sounds each time a key is depressed. People vary in their expectations of the 'feel' of a keyboard. Some like 'clicky' keyboards that offer a resistance when a key is pressed. Others prefer a fairly 'dead' keyboard that is almost silent. All this may sound like hair splitting but if you touch-type, have been used to a typewriter or have used a particular keyboard before, the question of the 'feel' of the keyboard is really important. I have had recent experience of this. Having just bought a new computer set-up, I struggled for some months to get used to the keyboard that goes with it.

In the end, I had to pay for a new one because the one supplied with the outfit was just too 'rubbery' and unresponsive. If you can, try out a number of keyboards before you settle on any particular one. Fortunately, keyboards are not particularly expensive and you can sometimes negotiate with a supplier as to the make and model that you buy with your computer. This only applies, of course, to desktop computers. With laptops, notebooks and palmtops (discussed below), you are stuck with the keyboard that comes with the machine. This is all the more reason why you should try before you buy.

The mouse

A mouse is a small unit attached by cable to the CPU. It can be moved around a desk top via a small ball in its base and is used as a 'pointer' in some computer programs. Such programs use what is known as a 'graphical user interface' (GUI). This means that you use the mouse to 'point' to menu items or small 'pictures' on the screen. Such a way of working is thought by many to be an easier one that using the keyboard. The Windows environment, described below, relies heavily on the use of a mouse, as do many drawing and graphics programs. Most computers today come ready supplied with a mouse. If your computer does not, you are advised to buy one.

Monitor

Currently, most computers come with a colour, VGA or Super VGA monitor. VGA stands for 'video graphics array' (commonly misquoted as 'video graphics adapter') – a standard of screen which replaced earlier EGA and MDA screens (see the Glossary for an explanation of these terms). Some people argue that mono (or black and white) screens are adequate or even preferable for wordprocessing. I often think that these debates are like the ones that occurred when colour televisions first became available. At that time, some people said they preferred black and white. In the end, a clear, colour monitor really does make a difference. While you can manage with a mono screen, you are most likely to prefer a colour one and the differences can go beyond simple preference. A colour screen allows you to allocate certain textual changes to certain colours. For example, you may want all italicized text to show up on your screen as red and all bold characters to be light blue and so on. Once you have allocated colours in this way, you are able to see at a glance any changes that you have made to your work on the screen.

For most wordprocessors, the default (or preset) background screen colour is blue with white text. You are usually free to change this setting and I have found that a dark blue background with yellow text is easy on the eye. You may prefer other settings.

Computing Tip 5

Copy protect your program disks

On all 3½" disks, there is a small piece of plastic sitting in a 'window' at the top of the disk. If you 'open' the window, the disk cannot be written to; it can only be read by your computer. Open all the windows on your program disks to avoid accidentally writing over them.

DESKTOP COMPUTERS

The name 'desktop' is fairly self-explanatory. The desktop computer is the one which sits on top of your desk and is, by and large, a fixture. It comprises the full size versions of the keyboard, monitor and CPU and is not very portable. There are a few 'miniature' desktop machines which are movable but the whole idea of the desktop is that it remains in one place for much of the time. The advantages of the desktop machine are that they usually offer an excellent keyboard and a very high quality monitor. While you may prefer to use a portable computer for your 'main' computer, it will be a long time before such machines can match the monitor quality of desktop machines. Also, portable computers nearly always offer a compromise on their keyboards. In order to enable them to be portable, the keyboard layout on the portable is often cramped and in a different layout to its desktop companion. Many senior health professionals use a desktop computer at work and a portable computer to work at home or on the move.

Working with a desktop computer

There are certain considerations to be made when using a desktop computer on a regular basis. These include the following:

- Position your computer carefully. You need to consider where you place your monitor in relation to a window. If you have the window behind you, you may find it difficult to read the screen.
- Check your seating position. Two medically related problems are common with computing: bad posture and repetitive strain injury (caused by fast and repetitive movements of the hands and fingers). The former can be avoided by paying attention to how you site your keyboard and monitor. The latter can be avoided by use of a rubber pad that sits in front of the keyboard and on which you rest your wrists. Such pads are available from computer accessory suppliers. It also helps if you break up the periods that you spend at the keyboard. It is the repetition of hand movements that causes the problems. If you can, take lots of breaks and work on a variety of tasks at the keyboard. If you have to do a lot of 'typing', break off occasionally to do some 'housekeeping' tasks on the computer. These are discussed in Chapter 4.
- Make sure that there is sufficient air flow around both your computer and (if you use one) your laser printer. Some components in some computers can heat up considerably. Laser printers also need a reasonable amount of ventilation.
- Consider the noise factor if you use a dot matrix printer. Many such printers can make considerable noise when they are in action. Make sure that this noise is not irritating people around you.
- Think carefully about lighting. Uplighting is usually preferable to a down-facing lamp as it causes less reflection on the monitor screen. If you are working near a window, do not sit with the window behind you but position the screen at right angles to the window. This, again, will help to cut down on reflections on the screen.
- Try various permutations of seating, lighting and positioning until you hit on the most comfortable and practical one for you.

LAPTOP COMPUTERS

The laptop computer is what it says: a portable computer that can, in theory, be used on your lap. In practice, laptops are usually a bit too heavy to be used in this way. They do, however, have all the functions of the desktop computer, housed in a box that can be easily transported.

They are heavier than their relatives, notebook computers, described below. Because notebook computers are becoming much cheaper to buy, laptops have become real bargains. It is sometimes possible to buy a fully functioning, portable laptop computer for less than the price of an equivalent desktop machine.

Laptops are not really suitable for carrying long distances. They are handy if you travel by car and want a portable computer that is not too expensive. If you plan to carry your computer with you when you travel, you are better advised to consider buying a notebook computer.

THE NOTEBOOK

The notebook is the ideal portable computer. It is much lighter than a laptop (about 5–7lbs in weight) and can be carried in a briefcase. The most common versions, at the moment, have black and white screens but many are now available with colour screens.

The notebook keyboard is sometimes a little cramped and you may find the layout is a little different to that of the desktop variety. This can cause problems for touch-typists. On the notebook computer that I use, for example, the cursor keys are not in the 'usual' position and I frequently find myself sending the cursor in the wrong direction. Check on the keyboard layout of the notebook computer you plan to buy, before you buy it. A small detail like this can make a lot of difference in using the machine.

All notebooks offer both battery and mains sources of power. One of the main areas of research in portable computing is centred around producing batteries that last longer. At the moment, the average time span of one charging of a notebook battery is about 2–3 hours. It is to be hoped that the figure will be tripled within the next couple of years.

If you travel with a notebook computer, you should have little trouble with Customs as long as you are prepared to show evidence of ownership and are also prepared to switch the machine on and show it working.

Working with a notebook

There are certain considerations you should bear in mind when working with a notebook computer on a regular basis. These include:

- Always back up your work to a floppy disk.
- Write your name on the bottom of the computer using an indelible pen.
- Stick a business card or other label inside the carrying case.
- Buy a couple of spare batteries. Then you can have one in your notebook and one being recharged.
- Buy an extra power lead. If you use your notebook at home and at work, use one of the leads at home and the other at work.
- Drain the battery regularly. Most notebooks use NiCad batteries which 'remember' the point at which you recharge them. If you recharge them when they are still 'half full', you will not be able to use them for very long before they run down. Instead, once a month, leave your computer switched on overnight and drain the battery completely. Then recharge the battery.
- To economize on battery use, turn the screen light down and consider working in 'reverse video'. Thus, instead of working with a white background and black characters on the screen, you work with a black background and white characters. Most notebooks allow you to change this setting through a 'set-up' program.
- If you travel with your notebook buy a good-sized 'weekend' bag. Use this in place of the bag that was supplied with your notebook. A larger bag will allow you to pack extra disks, an extra battery (if necessary) and any paperwork and books that you might need. If you fly with your computer, you will need to buy a case that will allow you to keep within the 'carry on' luggage limit. This will still allow you to buy a larger case than the one supplied with the computer.
- Give some consideration to how you sit in relation to your notebook computer. If you have to work in a hotel room, for example, it is tempting to sit or lay on the bed to do your work. This will quickly cause considerable physical discomfort. Remember the principles of seating and positioning from the earlier section on working with a desktop computer and think carefully about how you site your notebook. It is tempting, because a notebook computer is so small and light, to skimp on these sorts of details. If you do, you are likely to feel the consequences the next morning, when you wake up with a stiff neck and uncomfortable shoulders.

Example software: **LapLink Pro (Travelling Software)**

Many people work on more than one computer at different times. A number of health professionals will use a computer at home to work on projects, essays or lesson plans and then want to polish them up on the machine at work. Managers may use a notebook computer when they are travelling and then use a desktop computer back at base. A problem arises when there is a need to transfer information from one to the other. Traditionally, this has been done by swapping disks. With the development of notebooks and laptops that have larger hard disks, this is by no means an easy option. The best option lies with LapLink Pro.

This professionally packaged product comes complete with everything you need to transfer data from one computer to another. At one level, you simply plug in the leads, install the software and then 'pipe' your files from one to the other. The program is extremely easy to set up and the transfer rate is very speedy. This certainly beats the older disk-to-disk method.

LapLink can be used as a back-up system for backing up your data files to floppy disks or to another hard disk. It also has an impressive modem transfer capability where files can be transferred between PCs anywhere in the world. This system makes use of a modem and a telephone line. But, more cleverly still, the program also allows you to 'take control' of a distant computer and to collect files on that distant machine. This will be particularly useful for the manager or educator who has left a file at work and cannot drive in and pick it up. He or she simply calls up the work computer and downloads the file into his or her own desktop or notebook.

Help is always at hand with LapLink although you won't need much of it. Once you have read through the clearly written handbook and installed the program, the rest is very straightforward. It is a simple matter of comparing, side by side, the directories of two machines on screen at the same time. From those dual trees, you can pick and choose the files that you want to send or collect. It is also possible to 'spring clean' a distant computer – a task that some people may find more agreeable in the evening, away from work.

The program not only lets you work with data files but is quite happy dealing with program files too. You simply select a directory or a set of files to transfer and press a couple of keys. You then sit back and watch the program speedily sending the files to your other computer. The program is compatible with a very wide range of personal computers and also with a considerable number of modems. It does nothing to the files that you transfer so no 'unzipping' or other sort of adaptation is necessary once you have transferred files in this way. It also offers you a full statistical analysis of both of your computers. In this way, you are always able to tell how much room you have on either or both computers.

| Computing Tip 6 | **Keep your directory plan simple**

If possible, stick to 'one level' of directories. In other words, keep your wordprocessor in one directory, your spreadsheet in another and your data in another. Avoid layers of directories. These slow down your computer and make data difficult to find. |

Example software: **Battery Watch Pro (Travelling Software)**

If you use a portable computer – a laptop or a notebook – you are likely to find Battery Watch Pro useful. The thing that you don't want to do with a portable is to run the battery flat while you are working on important data. This program cuts down the chances of your doing this.

Battery Watch Pro can run in either a DOS or a Windows environment. It functions as a 'terminate and stay resident' program – which allows it to be 'popped up' over other programs.

Battery Watch Pro monitors your battery. By pressing ALT-SHIFT-B, you can call up a screen which tells you how much time you have left to work, using your battery. Alternatively, you can have a small digital 'clock' showing in the top right hand corner of the screen. This ticks away and lets you know how much longer you have. I liked the idea of this but found it unnerving in practice. I found myself becoming obsessed with clock-watching and imagining how much longer I could go on working.

Battery Watch Pro can be customized to support 50 popular laptops and notebooks – an improvement of 11 portables over the previous version of the program. Installation is simple. You insert the single disk into the drive of your computer, type INSTALL and the whole thing is unloaded onto your hard disk.

The tune-up feature of the program allows for even more accuracy in timing. It keeps track of how a person has used the portable computer over the last ten charges. It then assigns a 'time limit' to its clock, based on an average of those ten charges. The program also includes a 'deep discharge' feature which enables you to quickly drain your NiCad battery completely for recharging. With NiCad batteries, it is important that they are fully discharged before being recharged. Too frequent a recharging of a partially charged battery means that you are left with less battery power. A frequently charged battery will run out quickly.

Help for the program is available through the usual F1 function key and the package is completed by an easy to read and slim manual. There is not a lot to get to grips with. You simply install the program and forget it until you need to know the status of your battery.

PALMTOP COMPUTERS

Palmtops are the smallest computers of all. There is now a range of 'pocket sized' computers that can be used as personal organizers and for storing names and addresses and other data. They rarely have keyboards on which you can touch-type but they are, nevertheless, 'real' computers. Many are now PC compatible and you may want to use one of these as a replacement for your diary. Remember, though, that all the principles about backing up data from a hard disk to a floppy (discussed throughout this book) apply to palmtop computers too. If you do use a palmtop as a diary, your whole 'life' is contained within it. If you accidentally wipe off your next year's appointments, you are likely to find your life disrupted quite considerably. Make sure that at any given time you have a back-up of everything that is contained in your 'computer diary'. This point alone is enough to make some people feel that computer diaries are more bother than they are worth. In the end, many people return to the more simple approach of keeping a 'real' diary.

MODEMS

A modem is the means by which you can communicate between two or more computers via a telephone line. Technically, it is a *modulator–*

*dem*odulator, which allows the digital signals of the PC to be transmitted over the telephone. A modem can be either a stand-alone unit which plugs into the back of the computer or it can be on a card which is plugged into a free expansion slot, inside the case of the computer. To use a modem, you need the following:

- the modem itself;
- the software that allows you to use the modem;
- a telephone socket or a 'splitter' that allows you to use both a telephone and the modem from the same plug.

Modems can be used for a range of communication activities, including, at least, the following:

- sending electronic 'letters' to other people, through a system known as E Mail;
- sending data files to colleagues;
- transferring data to or from bulletin boards – electronic 'noticeboards' that allow people who are interested in a particular topic to communicate with each other;
- downloading shareware and public domain software;
- sending faxes direct from the computer;
- remotely operating another computer – your computer at work from your computer at home, for example;
- getting information from a range of databases. There are, for example, a number of medically oriented bibliographic databases that can be accessed via modems;
- checking airline timetables and bookings;
- sending files and data 'back to base' from a portable or notebook computer, whilst on the move;
- communicating with various electronic information services such as CompuServe.

A modem is a valuable addition to most computer set-ups. On the other hand, the installation of a modem means that your computer is no longer a totally closed system. The fact that you can call up data from other sources means that your computer may be at risk from computer viruses. For this reason, it is recommended that any data that is downloaded (or brought into your computer from an external source) is first screened by a virus checking program. This is particularly important when a computer is left on all of the time, with the modem always activated.

OTHER ADD-ONS

Apart from modems, there are various other things you can add on to your computer. This applies whether it is a desktop, laptop or notebook.

First, you may want to use a scanner. A scanner lets you import graphics and some forms of typescript into the computer via the appropriate software. Scanners are either hand-held or desktop. The technology is not yet available for scanners to reliably copy handwriting but good quality optical character recognition (OCR) software can usually make a reasonable job of typewritten and printed documents. Scanning is a slow process and is demanding of RAM (memory) and hard disk space. It cannot be relied on as a routine way of transferring data from one medium to another. Interestingly enough, if you have a large amount of interview, report or other data to transfer to your computer, it is still worth considering paying a copy typist to type it in. Sometimes the simplest solutions are the best ones.

You can also add on another, portable, hard disk unit. These come in small boxes that plug into the back of your computer. Such units are an ideal way of adding a hard disk to a notebook computer or as a method of transporting data from one place to another. If, for example, you use one desktop computer at work and another at home, it may be worthwhile investing in one of these portable hard disk packages. They can also be used as back-up units for backing up the contents of your hard disk.

Finally, you can send faxes via your computer. Some types of software allow you to send the fax direct from the screen. In this case – at your end, at least – no paper is involved. You simply use the keyboard to type your letter or document and then the software sends the message to the other person's fax machine in the normal way.

CD-ROM

The CD-ROM offers a method of retrieving large amounts of data from a compact disk. The initials stand for 'Compact Disk: Read Only Memory'. Thus, although data can be read into your computer from the compact disk, you cannot write new data to the disk. The CD-ROM player plugs into the back of your computer and software allows you to read screenfulls of data. Alternatively, you can have a CD-ROM drive slotted or built into your main computing unit. Some CD-ROM players for computers also play audio compact disks. When you are not using the machine for calling up data, you can use it to play music. While compact disks can store huge amounts of data (usually up to 650Mb per disk), access time to the disks is slower than to the fastest hard disks. On the other hand, the huge storage capacity makes them ideal for storing catalogues of bibliographic information, which is likely to be of value to many health care professionals. Many companies which specialize in the recording of bibliographic information offer subscription schemes whereby you receive updated disks every month or quarter. This is usually only an option for organizations rather than for individuals, as subscription rates are understandably high. Examples of journal listings on CD-ROM of interest to health care professionals are identified in Chapter 6 and are available from Microinfo Ltd, CD-ROM Division, PO Box 3, Omega Park, Alton, Hampshire GU34 2PG.

PRINTERS

The output from a personal computer is usually to a printer. There are three types of printer in use at the moment. These are:

- the dot matrix printer;
- the ink-jet printer;
- the laser printer.

The dot matrix printer uses a square matrix of nine or 24 'pins' which are inked by a ribbon and used in various formations to produce characters on the page. Nine pin printers typically produce a fairly 'grainy' output that is similar to a traditional typewriter. They are, however, the cheapest printers on the market and they can be picked up as considerable bargains. They are slower than the other sorts and tend to be noisy in operation.

The ink-jet printer works by squeezing ink through a tiny nozzle straight on to the paper. Although this sounds an unlikely arrangement, the output is nearly always excellent. Ink-jet printers are quiet to run, reasonably inexpensive and their output is of a much higher quality than that obtained from a dot matrix. These are the ones to go for if you are looking for a high quality printer for home use.

Laser printers offer the highest quality output of all. They are nearly always larger than ink-jet or dot matrix printers and more expensive. However, prices are generally falling all the time and the output from a laser printer is excellent. The best laser printers produce text that is almost indistinguishable from 'real printing'.

Apart from the initial outlay for the printer itself, you need to consider the running costs. All that you need to buy for a dot matrix printer is the occasional ribbon. It is impossible to say how long ribbons last because that depends on the model and on your level of use. Suffice it to say that a dot matrix ribbon usually lasts much longer than do the disposables for the other two sorts of printers. Usually, too, ribbons are fairly cheap.

The ink-jet printer uses a disposable cartridge of ink which does not normally last for very many pages of printing. There are kits available for refilling these cartridges but reports of these are variable and many people find that they have to buy complete cartridges each time that the output begins to get faint. Laser printers have two replaceable parts. First, the toner cartridge has to be replaced at intervals. These can vary in the number of pages that they allow you to print over quite a large range. Smaller toner cartridges may have to be replaced every 1000 copies whilst larger ones run to 5000 or more copies. Toner cartridges are usually considerably more expensive than ink-jet cartridges and very much dearer than dot matrix ribbons. In a laser printer, too, at some point, the drum within the machine has to be changed. This is a fairly rare occurrence but is expensive when it does happen.

Almost all dot matrix printers can handle both single sheets of paper and 'continuous' paper – paper that is perforated and runs continuously through the printer. Some ink-jet printers also allow you to use continuous paper but all laser printers only use single sheets. The speed of the laser printers means that not being able to use continuous paper is no handicap. And the relative speeds of the different machines can vary greatly. Here is an example from my own experience.

A few years ago, I used a nine pin dot matrix printer. At that time, to print out a 400 page book manuscript meant setting the printer up to run overnight with continuous paper. If I set it up to run from seven in the evening, it usually finished printing at about nine the next morning. Today, I use a laser printer and can print off a 400 page manuscript in about an hour.

If you want speed and quality, the laser printer is the printer of choice. If you want quality and economy, the ink-jet may be the answer. If you want economy of both initial outlay and of running costs, the dot matrix printer is the one to buy.

WHAT SORT OF COMPUTER SHOULD YOU BUY?

Taking all the issues above into account, the following guidelines can be laid down for buying a computer for home or light professional use:

- It should be IBM compatible.
- It should have a hard disk.
- It should be expandable. You should consider buying a computer whose main processing chip can easily be updated.
- It should have a monitor and keyboard that suit you.
- It should have sufficient RAM (random access memory) to allow you to use modern programs. As computers develop, so the RAM requirements grow.
- If you are going to do graphics work of any kind, it should have a colour monitor.
- It should be capable of running Windows, if you want it to have a degree of 'future proofing'.

FURTHER READING

Howard, W. (1991) *PC Magazine Guide to Notebook and Laptop Computers*, Ziff-Davis Press, Emeryville, California

If you use a computer, you are likely to be interested in laptops and notebooks. Both offer the power of a desktop computer with the convenience of the jumbo A4 pad of feint and margin. Bill Howard's *PC Magazine Guide to Notebook and Laptop Computers* offers you all you are ever likely to need to know about the topic. Much more than that, it is also thoroughly readable. It is a rare event that you find yourself reading a computer manual like a novel. But this author offers a style that must be a first in the computer world.

The book is exhaustive in its coverage. Beyond the obvious definitions of laptops and notebooks, the book offers you a blow-by-blow account of how and why you should make your choice.

The early chapters are likely to be useful to anyone who knows little about computers. They offer a very straightforward and clear account of the innards of any computer. They also help you to choose whether you need a desktop, a laptop or a notebook.

Next, the book offers useful advice about buying your computer. While not all the advice travels (the book is American), much of it does. It highlights the differences between buying through the post and in the High Street shops. Best of all, it does not offer one view of all this but always highlights all the pros and cons.

Later chapters deal with setting up your machine, working with it on the move and using a modem. Again, the detail becomes intriguing and although it is more than you are likely to need, it is always likely to be useful reference material. The final chapters discuss software and utilities that you can add on to your computer.

3 Buying and using a personal computer

So far, we have discussed the various considerations you should make when thinking about buying a personal computer. This chapter addresses the question of where and how to buy one.

CHANGING FROM A PCW

The Amstrad PCW (a computer, printer and wordprocessing package) was a popular buy for many health care professionals. The PCW was many people's introduction to computing and, for wordprocessing, still represents fairly good value for money. However, the price of personal computers has dropped dramatically in the last few years and many people are either trading up to PCs or buying them in the first place. If you are changing from a PCW to a PC, you will have to relearn a new keyboard and may want to think about changing your wordprocessing program. The PCW comes complete with the LocoScript wordprocessor. Many people also used the wordprocessor called Protext. Both are available in a personal computer format (you cannot simply swap machines and keep the software that you used with the PCW).

Both programs have a wide range of features and are good wordprocessors in their own right. There are, however, more comprehensive wordprocessors with more features. Also, neither LocoScript nor Protext (at the time of writing) will run under Windows. You may want to consider switching not only your computer but also your wordprocessor. Do not simply swap machines and stay with the wordprocessor because it seems to be the obvious thing to do. It may be. Equally, it may not be. While you are upgrading your hardware, you may also want to do the same with your software. Remember, too, that when you change from a

PCW to a PC, you will have to arrange for all of your data files to be converted into a format that can be read by your personal computer. There is a standard format for switching data from machine to machine, know as the ASCII (pronounced 'asky') format. This is an international data format that most computers can recognize and which most word-processors and other software programs can read. If you use an early PCW, you will also have to have all of your data files transferred to larger disks. The early PCWs used a non-standard 3" disk. Most PCs use the 3½" disk as standard.

POTENTIAL USER CHECKLIST

There are numerous questions to ask yourself, your friends and your dealer before you buy a computer. Here are some of them:

- How much money do you have to spend on computing equipment? Remember that you will need to buy both a computer and a printer. Remember, too, that companies rarely indicate a total price in their adverts: you usually have to add on VAT.
- What will you use your computer for? Wordprocessing rarely needs the power and capacity that desktop publishing does. If you are only going to wordprocess, do you need a state of the art machine?
- How much do you know about computers? Could you take advice from other people? Be wary of asking too many people: find someone whose advice you trust and stick to that person. It's easy to be overwhelmed.
- Do you need two types of floppy drive? If you are likely to use older programs or work with data stored on larger disks, it may be worth getting a machine with a 5¼" drive as well as a, now standard, 3½".
- Is speed important? If so, you are likely to need a 486 machine. Check that the hard disk times are also fast. The speed of the processor can be 'lost' in a computer that has a slow hard disk.
- What size hard disk do you need? Think of a number and then double it. You almost always end up filling the hard disk that you get, whatever the size you buy. Think very big when you plan to buy a hard disk.

- Are you going to work with graphics and diagrams? If so, you may want to consider a larger screen than the normal 14″. This will, of course, add further cost to your set-up.
- Will you need training? If you are completely new to computing, it may be worth investing in either an evening class before you buy your computer or an intensive training course in the software that you plan to use.
- What software will you be using? Will it work easily with the computer that you have in mind? Windows-based programs often take up very large amounts of hard disk. Make sure your hard disk is big enough to cope.
- How much memory do you want your computer to have? Like the hard disk issue, you can rarely have too much memory – especially if you plan to use Windows.
- What sort of printer do you want and what sort can you afford? Whilst a laser printer offers the highest quality print-out of all, ink-jet printers are much cheaper and can produce very high quality printing. Laser printers also cost more to run.
- Do you need a desk or table to accommodate your computer? Many of the ready-to-buy computing desks look fine in an office but not in a home. Think carefully about the new furniture that you need to buy. As ever, it is wise to negotiate these sorts of issues with the people with whom you live. Computer furniture may be functional but it rarely conforms to what most people would think of as 'household furniture'.

HOW TO FIND THE RIGHT DEALER

You can buy computers in many High Street stores. The ones to look for are those that only sell computers. The general electrical and computing stores tend to be less competitive in their prices and their staff tend not to be so well informed. You cannot expect people who work in general stores to be computing experts – although some are.

General stores often advertise what appear to be bargains by quoting 'listed' prices and then discounting these. If you buy computing magazines, however, you will soon discover that these are rarely the bargains they seem. On the other hand, the big advantage of buying in a large electrical chain store is that you can usually depend on good service if you have to return goods. They usually have a reputation to defend.

Specialist computer shops are often the ones in which the computer experts work. They tend, though, to be more expensive than the companies that sell through the post. If you are not sure of what you want, they may be the place to start learning. As a general rule, though, if you are going shopping for a computer, take a friend who knows about computers with you.

Computing Tip 7

Keep your machine switched on

If at all possible, keep your computer switched on for as long as possible. The thing that helps to wear it out quickest is frequently switching it on and off. When you first get your computer, try to leave it on continuously for 72 hours. Most faults show up during this period. If it survives this initial 72 hours, it is likely to give you pain free work for a considerably longer period. The average life of a computer is about 4–5 years.

Superstores

There are an increasing number of computer supermarkets opening in the UK. Popular for some years in North America, such stores offer a wide range of computers, software and peripherals. They are not normally as competitive as dealers who sell through the post (see below) but the big advantage of the superstore is that you can see what it is you are buying before you commit yourself.

BUYING THROUGH THE POST

Many computers are sold direct to the customer and some companies have become famous for both their level of customer service and for their reasonable prices: Dell and Elonex are but two examples. Generally speaking, buying through the post is nearly always a cheaper option than buying from a dealer. Overheads are lower and there is no middle man in the deal. Most of the larger and many of the smaller companies advertise regularly in the computer magazines and it is worth buying a few of these to compare prices.

The main point about buying in this way is that you need to know what it is you want to buy. You will not be able to try out the keyboard, you will have to specify, exactly, what sort of machine you want and you will not see it until it arrives. On the other hand, if you do know what you want, buying direct is likely to offer you the best value for money.

When you buy a computer through the post you can also buy the level of service that you need, from on-site to back-to-base. You can usually specify the length of such an agreement and buy extra years of cover if you require it. It is usually better to buy as lengthy a service agreement as you can afford.

If you are ordering over the phone, you may want to get various quotes for prices from various companies. To do this, you need to be able to tell each company exactly what you want. The following checklist identifies the information that you need to have in front of you when you ask for a quote:

- model of computer;
- main chip (386, 486, etc.);
- speed in MHz;
- floppy drives (720k, 1.44Mb, etc.);
- hard disk size;
- standard memory (RAM);
- additional memory required;
- operating system included (DOS? DOS with Windows? None?);
- other software 'bundled' with the computer;
- mouse included in the price?
- type of casing: desktop, tower?
- details of warranty;
- details of service agreement;
- price with VAT;
- cost of any other extras;

- delivery charge;
- availability and delivery.

RENTING AND LEASING

Some health care professionals work as independent practitioners. If you are self-employed, you may want to rent or lease a computer. Renting is usually a short term option and is much more expensive. You may want to rent a computer for a week or two to type up the final draft of a dissertation, thesis or research report. Leasing, although cheaper, commits you to a three, four or five year contract. There are two important points about leasing. First, you can normally offset the whole of the amount that you spend on leasing against tax: a leased computer is counted as a 'consumable' for tax purposes. Second, a leasing agreement can enable you to upgrade your computer on a regular basis.

Read any agreement carefully before you sign either a rental or a leasing agreement. Check the amount that you are being charged for the hardware and check the servicing agreement. Some companies offer you 'free' servicing for the first year of the agreement and then ask you to pay a yearly sum for further servicing. Check, too, whether or not servicing will be 'on-site'. There is nothing worse than having to pack your computer back up in its original containers and ship it back to the company.

BUYING SECONDHAND

There are not many things that can go wrong with a computer as there are relatively few moving parts. The most fragile things are the drives, particularly the hard disk drive. Secondhand computers can be real bargains but there are two main problems with buying a secondhand machine. First, you are nearly always buying old technology: people usually sell their computers to upgrade. This may be no problem if you plan to use the computer for straightforward tasks such as word-processing. Second, people often have an inflated idea about what their computer is worth. One glance through any computer magazine that has a 'For Sale' section will confirm this. Many of the machines in these columns are more expensive than the new computers that are advertised by dealers. Be prepared to do some haggling. Also, take a knowledgeable friend with you to look at a secondhand computer. Ask to see the computer up and running. Then, check the following:

- Make sure that all the keys on the keyboard work. Press them, systematically, and watch the reaction on the screen. Obviously, every key should work and should produce the right reaction.
- Try out the disk drive(s). Put a disk into the floppy drive and make sure that the computer can 'read' the disk.
- Having taken a program with you on a floppy disk, run the program on the computer and make sure that everything works as it should.
- Look at the overall cleanliness of the outside of the computer. Keyboards, for example, can become clogged up and this can lead to keys not working. Some authorities insist that you can wash a keyboard under the tap if it is dirty. I've never tried this and don't really recommend it.
- Ask to look inside the central computing unit. Have your knowledgeable friend check over the internal components. Also, check that the inside of the machine is reasonably clean.
- Identify what (if any) software is being sold with the computer. Check that all of this comes complete with the original manuals. If the manuals are not available, you may be buying pirated software.

Computing Tip 8	**Keep a back-up of your AUTOEXEC.BAT and CONFIG.SYS files on a separate disk (these terms are explained in Chapter 4)**
	Always have a copy of your AUTOEXEC.BAT and CONFIG.SYS files on a floppy disk. If your hard disk fails or those files become corrupt on your hard disk, you will need such a disk to reboot your computer (as long as you have formatted that disk with the command FORMAT /s first). In an emergency, you can use your original DOS disks to reboot but a 'standby' disk is preferable.

CONSUMABLES

In this case, 'consumables' refers to all those parts of computing that are used up over a period of time. Typically, a list of consumables includes the following:

- ink, ribbons or cartridges for your printer;
- paper;
- floppy disks.

You can sometimes buy ink, ribbons or cartridges in bulk and thus save money. A cartridge for a laser printer can cost up to £100 to replace. With a laser printer, you also have to replace the drum, inside the printer, at fairly well spaced out intervals. This adds another cost to running the machine.

Paper for computers comes in various types. Dot matrix printers and some ink-jets can often run 'continuous paper'. This is the sort that comes in the form of a continuous length that is perforated between sheets and at the sides. The continuous paper is pulled or pushed through the printer. After you have finished printing, you tear the pages apart. This approach to printing means that you do not have to feed single sheets into your machine. You simply set up the printer and leave it to finish the job. You quickly get used to tearing the sheets apart (a few pages at a time) cleanly. On the other hand, the fact that you have used continuous paper is usually fairly obvious. Even 'microperforated' paper has a slightly serrated edge left on it after it has been separated.

Some dot matrix and most ink-jets can work with what is rather clumsily called a 'cut-sheet feeder'. This is a contraption that fits on the printer (and is usually sold separately from it) which allows you to stack up a number of single sheets of paper at a time. These sheets then feed themselves through the printer, one at a time.

All laser printers only take single sheets of paper and you simply buy packets of copier or other paper. For high quality work, it is a good idea to buy 'heavy' paper. Conqueror Bond is an example of a good quality paper. For less important work and for drafts, you can use photocopier paper. It is worth shopping around for this. Prices vary widely and some of the best deals can be found in stationery cash and carry stores.

Floppy disk prices also vary widely. Most sorts of disks are reliable and you can often buy very large quantities at very low prices, through the post. If you are lazy and rich, you can buy preformatted disks which you can use straight out of the box. It is often a good idea to club together with friends to buy larger numbers of disks at a considerable discount.

STARTING OUT

Allow yourself time to get used to using a computer if the one you have bought is your first. Don't rush to unpack it and plug it in. Take time to read through the various introductory manuals. Very often, much of the initial setting up of the computer has already been done by the manufacturer and dealer. If you read through the introductory material you will be better able to judge what you need to do and what has already been done.

Then, once you have the machine up and running, allow yourself some more time to familiarize yourself with it. Allow a considerable amount of time to get the printer set up, in my experience, one of the most time consuming and frustrating aspects of computing. In my case, that frustration has usually been caused by my own impatience. The answers to most of the problems of setting up a computer system are in the manual. So, the first rule of computing is simple: **read the manual**. No one pretends that computer manuals are always well written but they nearly always show you the basic principles of setting up. Better still, get someone who knows about computers to be with you when you set it up. They have usually had experience of initial problems and will know how to sort them out. There is nothing worse than being stuck with a new computer that does not seem to want to work. If problems continue, ring the support line at the company which supplied the equipment: the people there will almost always be able to 'talk you through' the stages of setting up.

FURTHER READING

Nelson, K.Y. (1992) *Voodoo DOS*, Ventana Press, Chapel Hill, North Carolina

Once you have bought your computer, you need to be able to set it up and work with it. This strangely named book is just what you need. It offers a wide range of tips on starting up and working with DOS. More than that, it's also easy to read. The writer is a computer journalist of some years' experience and it shows in this excellent book. An entertaining as well as useful book.

4 Operating systems and housekeeping with the personal computer

Personal computing is more than just using programs. It is also concerned with making sure that the computer runs smoothly and about finding files when you need them. I had a colleague once who bought a new PC and immediately copied all his programs and all his data files straight onto his hard disk. This meant that all of the files were jumbled together in the main (or 'root') directory. As a result, it took him ages to find a particular file. It also meant that he could not easily erase a program, even if he wanted to. If all program and data files are stored on the hard disk together, it becomes impossible to know which files belong to which program. The answer is to learn some of the basics of housekeeping. In order to do that, it is also necessary to get to grips with the operating system. This chapter discusses housekeeping, operating systems and operating system utilities.

OPERATING SYSTEMS

You cannot simply load programs into a computer, whatever sort you decide to buy. First, you must load an operating system. An operating system acts as a sort of framework within which all your programs run. If you have a hard disk, the computer first looks on that for the essential operating system files before it allows you to load any programs. There are various operating systems available but still the most frequently used one is Microsoft's DOS (Disk Operating System).

Having an operating system is not an option. It is an essential part of working with a personal computer.

DOS

DOS (Disk Operating System) allows you to do a variety of things. First, it lets you run the computer. It is the means by which computer programs are run inside the computer. Second, it offers you a range of 'utilities': copying, backing up and deleting files, formatting (or preparing) disks so that they are ready to receive data, enabling the computer to recognize the disk drives and so on. DOS is run by a series of commands or instructions that you type when you see the prompt when you first turn on your computer. There are few short cuts here. You simply have to sit down with the manual or a 'how to do it' book and learn the basics of DOS commands. Whatever set-up you use and whether or not you use the shells and menuing systems described below, you are still going to have to encounter DOS commands at some stage in your computing career. DOS is not difficult to learn and it is essential that you slowly get to grips with the more common commands. You also need to know how to set up and run two essential files: AUTOEXEC.BAT and CONFIG.SYS. Your computer looks for these two files every time you turn it on and it is important that you have a basic understanding of what these files do and how you can modify them if necessary. It is also essential that you have back-up copies of these two files on a separate floppy disk, just in case something goes wrong with your original or hard disk. Without these files, the computer will not be able to run programs. Both of these files are discussed, in detail, in the manuals that are supplied with DOS. Many companies supply computers with DOS already installed on the hard disk and with simple AUTOEXEC.BAT and CONFIG.SYS files already in place. As you buy new programs, however, you are likely to want to make changes to either or both of them.

The two most frequently encountered DOS versions are MS-DOS by Microsoft and DR-DOS by Digital Research.

DOS shells and menuing systems

DOS is not always the simplest of systems to run. In order to call up your programs, you need to be able to find your way to the right directory and then you need to know the letters that fire up the program. There are a number of programs on the market that allow you to avoid DOS almost altogether. A simple menuing system lists your programs on the screen and then invites you to press a single button to start up a particular program.

With a shell program, you are also able to switch in and out of a program to work on other programs. For example, WordPerfect Office (described below) allows you to switch out of your wordprocessor into your database and return to where you left your wordprocessing. Shells also contain subprograms which allow you to copy, delete and back up files without having to use the DOS copy commands.

Shells and menu systems take some of the complexity out of personal computing although they are often frowned upon by some computer buffs who believe that everyone should master DOS commands. The point is, of course, that you must learn some of those commands. If anything goes wrong and your computer 'hangs' or stops, then you need to know how to rescue your programs and your data. On the other hand, it seems reasonable to make life simple from a day to day point of view. I know many of the DOS commands but I still use a shell program from which to launch my programs and to copy and back up files. This is simply because a shell is simpler and quicker to use than the DOS commands. Examples of commercially available menuing and shell systems include:

- Direct Access
- X Tree Gold
- WordPerfect Office
- MS-DOS
- DR-DOS
- Powermenu
- Windows
- Desqview

Various shareware versions of DOS shell menus are identified in Appendix 3 of this book. Shareware itself is discussed in Chapter 8.

Example software: **WordPerfect Office (WordPerfect UK)**

Office is a suite of programs that can help you to organize a variety of aspects of your working life and of your PC.

First, Office offers a simple menuing system. The menu can be edited to allow you to call up any number of programs at the touch of a button. You may, for example, designate the letter W to your wordprocessor. Then, from your menu screen, you simply press W to fire up your wordprocessor. The menu system can be set up so that it appears on the screen as soon as you turn on your computer. In this way, you can bypass the complications of the DOS operating system altogether. You can forget all about 'paths' and 'syntax' and use the menu to guide you through the computer. You can also use the menuing system on a network which should make this an attractive package for larger organizations.

Office also includes a very useful file management program which is also started from the menu screen. This system lists all your files in all your directories and subdirectories. By using the cursor to move through the files, you can move, delete, copy or erase any one or more of them. You can also use the file manager to do back-ups of your data files from your hard disk to floppies. You can choose to have your files listed in a straightforward, down the screen list or in the more familiar 'tree' format. You can also use the file manager to view the contents of particular files. If, for example, you are trying to find an essay you wrote about the nursing process, you simply move the cursor on to the file that you think might be the one and press 'Enter'. You are then able to scroll through the contents of the text file without having 'first' to load it into your wordprocessor.

Office also contains a simple text editor. You can use this to edit or rewrite those two essential files that you must have in your root directory: CONFIG.SYS and AUTOEXEC.BAT. The first file gets the computer up and running, the second takes you into the programs that you want to run. You cannot easily edit these files in a wordprocessor but you can in the program editor of Office. You can also use it for simple notes and memos.

Then, there is the appointments scheduler. This offers you a diary into which you can program all your appointments during the next few days, months or years. You can also draw up 'to do' lists with this part of the program. The program can also be set with a series of alarms to remind you of important events. The question arises, of course, as to whether or not you would want to keep your appointments on computer. As we have seen, many of us like to carry our appointment times around with us in a diary. Having them on computer means that you have to be at your computer to keep track of those appointments.

Office also contains a simple database program which is ideal for storing names and addresses or bibliographical references. The Office suite can be customized in all sorts of ways. You can set up a 'welcome' banner at the top of the opening screen. If you use a coloured screen you can change them to suit your particular needs and wants. The file manager can be modified to show lists of files, a tree structure or both of these together on two halves of the screen.

WINDOWS

Windows by Microsoft is neither an operating system nor a shell in the sense that WordPerfect Office is a shell. Windows is a program that lets you access most of the commands that drive your computer and access your programs through the use of 'icons' or tiny pictures on the screen. You point to these icons by using a mouse and this means that you avoid having to learn the DOS commands. Many people find this method of working quicker and easier to learn, although Windows operates much more slowly than does 'bare' DOS. Windows also allows you to 'multi-task' if you have a sufficiently powerful computer, which means that you can run a number of programs at once. For example, you may have your wordprocessor printing out a document 'in the background' whilst you are working on a spreadsheet. The term 'windows' refers to what you see on the screen when you work in this way. Each program that you call up appears in a small (or large) 'window' or square on the screen. You can resize these windows so that they are tiny or so that they occupy the whole of the screen.

Windows also operates with graphical user interface (GUI) which enables the use of clear graphics or pictures as part of the programs. One of the most important elements of a GUI program is that it allows for a 'what you see is what you get' (WYSIWYG) presentation. Thus, what you see on the screen is what gets printed out. This is not necessarily true with DOS programs. The text on the screen in a DOS wordprocessor may bear little resemblance to the text that is printed out, whilst a GUI program will show you all the details that are to be printed out, including bold, italics, large print and so on. Many people feel that both GUI and the 'what you see is what you get' formats make Windows a much more user-friendly environment.

Waddilove (1992) suggests ten stages in changing over from DOS to Windows:

1. Hardware

First, to run Windows at all, you need a certain type of personal computer. The latest version of DOS calls for at least a 286 processor and you are likely to need between 3Mb and 4Mb of RAM to run it successfully. Also, the program occupies a large amount of hard disk space so an 80–100Mb hard disk is to be recommended.

2. Configuration

Before you install Windows, you need to make sure that your AUTOEXEC.BAT file does not contain pop-up programs (or 'terminate and stay resident' programs) that might conflict with the running of Windows.

3. Installation

The installation of Windows is usually fairly straightforward and the first disk of the program contains a simple 'set-up' program that helps you to load automatically.

4. Fine tuning

Once Windows is loaded, you can check whether or not it will run with any disk caching programs that you have. A disk cache program helps other programs to run more quickly but some will work with Windows and some will not. After basic installation, you can check whether or not the ones that you have will work.

5. Customizing

Windows can be customized in various ways. Waddilove (1992) suggests at least the following options:

- altering the amount of space between the icons on the screen;
- modifying the width of the borders around the individual windows;
- changing the colour scheme and the 'wallpaper' that decorates the back of the screen;

- modifying the speed of the cursor movement when you use it with a mouse.

6. *DOS programs*

Windows usually checks to see what programs are on your hard disk as it is installing itself. When it finds a program, it incorporates its name into the icon system and offers you the chance to fire up the program from the program manager. Sometimes, though, DOS-based programs are missed at installation. At this stage, you can manually install DOS programs so that each of them has its own icon.

7. *Accessories*

Various 'add-ons' are available to work alongside and with Windows. As you get more used to Windows you may want to try some of these as many are available as shareware (the concept of shareware is discussed in Chapter 8 of this book). Also, various accessories are packaged with Windows. You get a simple wordprocessor called Write, a notebook program, a clock and a calculator. You may want to spend time getting to know these accessories. They are also a useful means of learning about the total concept of Windows.

8. *Windows programs*

More and more programs are being written specifically for the Windows environment. For example, the well-known wordprocessors WordPerfect and Word have both been rewritten to run in Windows although both are also still available as DOS-only applications. Again, you may want to add these to your collection of programs. One of the strengths of the Windows environment is that many programs written for Windows share a common user interface. That is to say that the screen and menu layouts are similar when you move between programs. Usually, the menu bar is at the top of the screen and once you have learned one Windows program, you will find subsequent ones easier to learn.

9. *Utilities*

One of the important utilities that is available for Windows are various font packages. The word font strictly refers to sets of print types. Increasingly, though, it is being used in a more general way to refer to 'typefaces'. Add-on font programs are available from third party suppliers to add interest to what you see on the screen and what is printed out.

10. Deleting DOS programs

If you are finally sold on Windows, you may, as a final step, want to delete your DOS-based programs altogether. My suggestion would be that if you do this, hang on to the disks in case, at a later date, you decide to switch back. Whilst Windows is certainly more attractive as a user-computer interface, it is also much slower. At the time of writing, I have found it prudent to stick with DOS. By the time this book appears in print, it seems likely that I will have had to convert to Windows – simply because almost all manufacturers of software appear to be producing Windows-based products at the expense of DOS-based ones. Only a longer term appraisal of the product will enable users to decide whether or not Windows really is the ideal environment.

WINDOWS OR DOS?

Should you run DOS-only programs, or should you go for DOS and Windows? One thing needs to be clear: you cannot simply choose one or the other. Whilst you can run programs under DOS, you also need DOS if you are going to run Windows. As we have seen, Windows is not an operating system – it sits 'on top' of DOS. There is a new operating system available, called OS/2, which can run both DOS and Windows programs and is more powerful than either. It does, however, call for a very powerful computer with a large hard disk and a large amount of memory.

If you choose to run Windows, you should bear in mind that Windows programs are almost always slower to run that those that run directly in DOS. To enable Windows to run at all, you need at least a 286 (and preferably a 386) computer and at least 2Mb of memory (and preferably at least 4Mb). Windows itself takes up a considerable amount of hard disk space, as do programs that run under Windows. So you will need a large hard disk.

On the other hand, the benefits of Windows are clear. You can run more than one program at once; you do not have to rely on obscure 'commands' to run programs – instead you use a mouse and simple pull-down menus. Also, you have the benefit of WYSIWYG – you can see almost exactly what your final document will look like on the screen.

Although Windows is fast becoming a standard, you need to think carefully before making the switch. If most of your computing involves straightforward text editing, then a DOS-based wordprocessing program may be all you need. At the moment, I have to admit that for wordprocessing, I prefer a DOS-based program. It allows me to work quickly, without taking my hands off the keyboard to work the mouse. On the other hand, if you plan to do a lot of desktop publishing, then a Windows program is probably just what you need. Also, just to complicate matters, it is worth remembering that you can still run most of your DOS-based programs from the Windows screen. Also, not all computer programs are written for Windows: a number are still available only as DOS-based programs.

In the end, it is quite possible to use a mixture of the two. There is no such thing as 'future proofing' in computing. New models and new programs are becoming available all the time. If you want to try to anticipate the future, however, you are probably best off getting Windows. After all, you will have the DOS system with the computer when you buy it. The Windows program is not expensive and having it will mean that you can work with Windows programs as well as DOS programs. If all this sounds like sitting on the fence, it is! At the time of writing, the market has not settled down sufficiently to say whether or not Windows will take over completely from the DOS environment, but it certainly looks as though it might.

If you are already familiar with DOS, however, you do not have to be in a great rush. If you have been working with a wordprocessing program for some time, you are likely to have built up considerable skill in using it. You are likely to have worked out how to use most of the functions that you need and will know where to find the other ones. If you change to a Windows environment (even though the layout of these programs is more straightforward), you are going to have to learn a new way of working. Add to that the fact that your new Windows wordprocessor will run more slowly and all this means that you need to be very sure about needing to change before you do so. In the end, like most things in life, it's up to you.

DESQVIEW

An alternative to Windows is Desqview by Quarterdeck. Desqview is a multitasking program that works with DOS-based applications and also with Windows. In fact, it is three programs in one, but more about that later. To run Desqview 386, you need a 386 or 486 computer and it is advisable to have more than 640k of RAM. There is, however, another version of Desqview for 286 computers.

The main Desqview program is both simple to install and easy to use. You install it onto your hard disk and, during installation, the program searches your hard disk for programs. From that search, Desqview automatically develops a menu system which includes those programs.

When you load Desqview, you are presented with that menu and from it, you start up the program that you need. When you want to switch to another program, you simply press ALT and back comes the menu. You are then free to load up your second (and third and subsequent) program(s), as required. Each program runs in a half-screen 'window' and you can switch between these windows (and thus between your programs) by tapping twice on the ALT key. If you don't like working in a window, you simply press ALT+Z and the current program fills the screen. When you next want to swap programs, pressing ALT takes you back to the menu.

Desqview offers you a simple-to-use way of working with a variety of programs and lets you switch between them in a few seconds. To work with large programs, quickly, you will need a fair amount of memory. If you do not have that memory, Desqview simply ships your programs out to disk and still lets you recall them but a little more slowly. Either way, you are saved the trouble of closing down one program simply to look at another. When you 'leave' a particular program, you are later 'returned' to exactly the spot that you left.

You can also do more sophisticated multitasking. Supposing, for example, your wordprocessor takes some time to print out a document and does not allow you to leave the program until you have finished printing. You, on the other hand, want to work on your database or spreadsheet program. Desqview allows you to do all this. You set your wordprocessor printing, then you call up your database or spreadsheet 'over' the wordprocessing program. Meanwhile, your document continues to be printed out 'in the background' and you are free to do other things.

The program is exceptionally flexible. You can set up 'macros' – sets of keystrokes that are later released by a single keypress. You may, for example, set one up that loads up three or four programs at a time. For the compulsive 'fiddler', Desqview is a real find. You can spend hours adjusting and modifying the program to suit your particular needs. On the other hand, if you just want to work, you can do that too.

One of the many clever things about Desqview is its ability to run two versions of the same program at the same time. Thus, you may be developing two diagrams, in two screens, at the same time and switching between them. This facility is particularly useful if you do a lot of editing of reports, research proposals, essays, chapters or books.

As suggested above, Desqview is three programs in one. The other two are the programs that are bundled with the main Desqview program. One is the famous memory manager, QEMM. Anyone who uses a 386 or 486 computer with more than 640k of memory will appreciate the need to use such a manager. DOS will only address 640k of RAM and QEMM is a program which allows you to use any memory above that ceiling. It also does much more. Through its 'Optimize' function, it analyses your upper memory (extended, expanded and 'high') and then loads any 'terminate and stay resident' programs that you are using (such as Sidekick) into upper memory, along with various device drivers. It also does this by making the most economical use of memory it can and runs through hundreds of permutations in order to free as much conventional memory for 'standard' programs. Like Desqview, QEMM is an extremely flexible program that can help you to make best use of your computer's memory. It works in conjunction with the third element in the package: Manifest.

Manifest is a separate program that analyses your computer's use of memory and then gives you a detailed report of it. Manifest is a valuable program for those in the know. Computer addicts who like to fine tune their computers will find Manifest a valuable addition to their armoury. Manifest also teaches you quite a lot about your computer and its memory.

WHAT IS 'HOUSEKEEPING'?

Housekeeping is the name given to the task of managing your files on your hard disk. From the day you buy your computer and set it up, you should get into the habit of making sure that you have organized and backed up your files. If you do not, you are either likely to erase some important ones or you will get in a mess.

Naming files

Whenever you create a datafile, you will have to give it a name, so that it can be stored on your disk or on floppies. You are allowed to use up to eight letters, then a full stop and then three more letters (known as an extension), to name any file. It is helpful if you use names that remind you of what is in the file. For example, MOTHER.LTR may be more useful as the name of a file containing a letter to your mother than would be the name Q232RT.AFG. There are, however, names that you must avoid because they are also the names of commands or files in the DOS operating system. These are the names that you must avoid as single file names, without extensions.

APPEND	DIR	KEYB	RESTORE
ASSIGN	DISKCOMP	KEYBUK	RMDIR
ATTRIB	DISKCOPY	LABEL	SELECT
BACKUP	ECHO	MD	SET
BREAK	ERASE	MKDIR	SHARE
CD	EXE2BIN	MODE	SHIFT
CHCP	EXIT	MORE	SORT
CHDIR	FASTOPEN	NLSFUNC	SUBST
CHKDSK	FDISK	PATH	SYS
CLS	FILES	PAUSE	TIME
COMMAND	FIND	PRINT	TREE
COMP	FOR	PROMPT	TYPE
COPY	FORMAT	RD	VER
COUNTRY	GOTO	RECOVER	VERIFY
CTTY	GRAFTABLE	REM	VOL
DATE	IF	RENAME	XCOPY
DEL	JOIN	REPLACE	

You must also avoid any spaces in between letters in your file names and you cannot use the tab key or the CTRL character whilst naming files. You can, however, use any of the following symbols in your names:

$ # & @ ! ( ) - _ { } ~ ^ `

You may, for example, want to use one of these as a reminder of a particular type of file. You might devise a system whereby all of your heath related files included the extension .###. For example, a letter that you have written to a GP asking him for permission to collect research data from his practice may be called PERMISS.###. Note, however, that you cannot use the following symbols in file names:

* + = [ ] ; : , / ? .

(except when the . is between the main file name and its extension). There are also other combinations of three letters that you cannot use, routinely, as file extensions because of their use in the DOS operating system. They are:

BAK EXE
BAS MSG
BAT SYS
COM TMP
DOC $$$

Managing files

You cannot simply copy files onto your hard disk from a floppy. If you do, they will all end up in what is called the 'root' directory. Instead, you need to arrange your files in separate 'subdirectories' that contain all of your files neatly stored away according to type or according to program. Subdirectories are a bit like the drawers in a filing cabinet. Each draw contains folders about different things. Also, each drawer contains 'cradles' that keep your papers in an order within each drawer. Thus, in organizing your files on a computer, you can have one level of subdirectories (the drawers of the filing cabinet) and then a second level of subdirectories 'underneath' each of the previous ones (the cradles within the drawers).

Here is an example. You may begin by creating four subdirectories on your hard disk. Those four will contain four types of files:

- wordprocessing files
- spreadsheet files
- database files
- datafiles

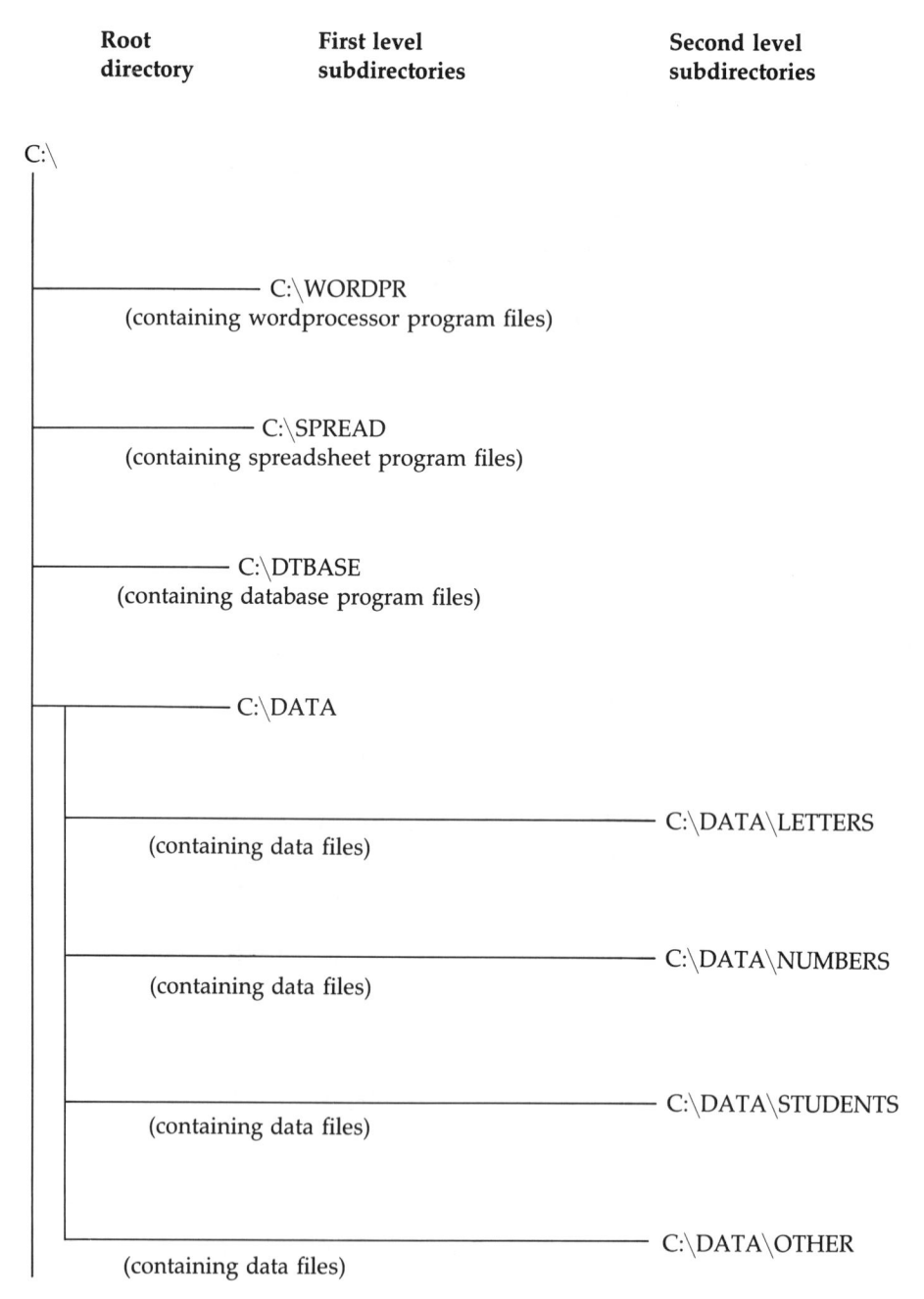

```
Root                First level              Second level
directory           subdirectories           subdirectories

C:\
 │
 ├──────── C:\WORDPR
 │         (containing wordprocessor program files)
 │
 ├──────── C:\SPREAD
 │         (containing spreadsheet program files)
 │
 ├──────── C:\DTBASE
 │         (containing database program files)
 │
 └──────── C:\DATA
           │
           ├──────────────────────────── C:\DATA\LETTERS
           │   (containing data files)
           │
           ├──────────────────────────── C:\DATA\NUMBERS
           │   (containing data files)
           │
           ├──────────────────────────── C:\DATA\STUDENTS
           │   (containing data files)
           │
           └──────────────────────────── C:\DATA\OTHER
               (containing data files)
```

Figure 4.1 Root directory and subdirectories on a hard disk.

You then copy your wordprocessing program into the subdirectory called WORDPR, your spreadsheet files into SPREAD and so on. Many programs create their own subdirectories when you install them onto your hard disk. The datafiles subdirectory (called DATA) contains any files that you create in your wordprocessing, spreadsheet or database programs.

Now the second level of subdirectories. You will not want to store all of your data files in the same subdirectory. You are likely to want to keep them grouped according to what sort of data they contain. Thus, beneath the DATA subdirectory, you create three more subdirectories, perhaps named as follows:

- LETTERS
- NUMBERS
- STUDENTS
- OTHER

It is in these subdirectories that you store your datafiles as you create them. Figure 4.1 illustrates the relationship between the root directory and the subdirectories that you have created. The row of letters and backslashes, in each case, is called the PATH – it leads you, via DOS commands, to the subdirectory in question. For example, this is what you would type to move from the root directory (c:\) to the data that contains your files about students. In this example, the letters 'CD' are the DOS command meaning 'change directory':

cd\DATA
cd\DATA\STUDENTS

Normally, when you first turn on your computer, you will find yourself in the root directory at the 'C prompt' (c:). In order to start your programs or to look at your datafiles, you first need to move to the appropriate subdirectories. The exception to this is if you have a PATH command in your AUTOEXEC.BAT file. The PATH command is a line in that file that looks something like this:

PATH c:\WORDPR;C:\SPREAD;C:\DTBASE;C:\DATA;

This commands tells the computer to 'look' in each of these directories for a file name that you type at the C prompt. Say, for example,

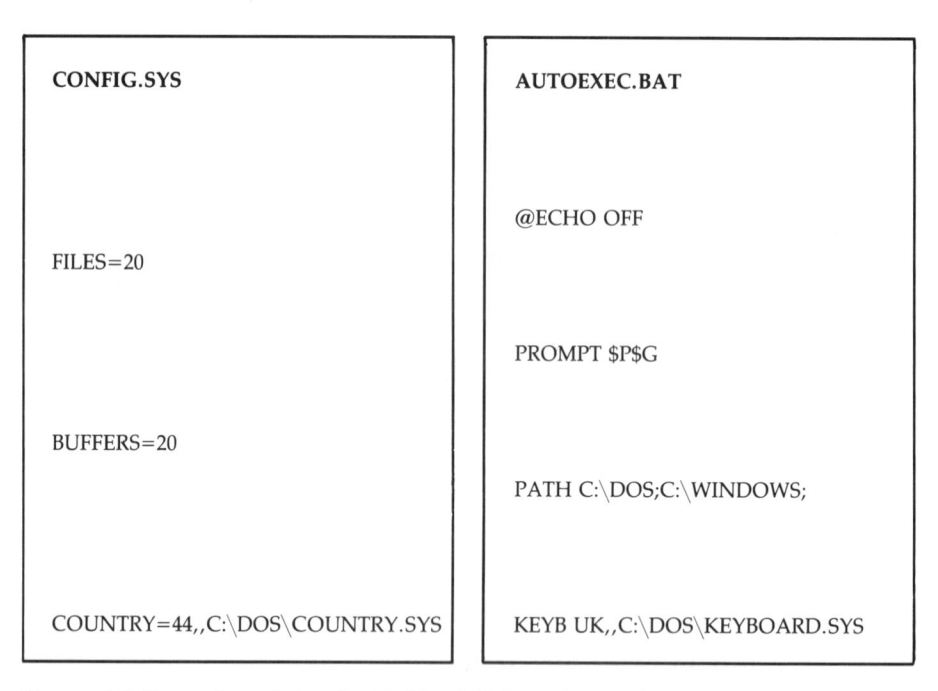

CONFIG.SYS	AUTOEXEC.BAT
FILES=20	@ECHO OFF
	PROMPT PG
BUFFERS=20	PATH C:\DOS;C:\WINDOWS;
COUNTRY=44,,C:\DOS\COUNTRY.SYS	KEYB UK,,C:\DOS\KEYBOARD.SYS

Figure 4.2 Examples of simple CONFIG.SYS and AUTOEXEC.BAT files.

your wordprocessing program (in the subdirectory, c:\WORDPR) is started by the letters WP. If you did not have a PATH command in your AUTOEXEC.BAT file, you would have to type the following commands, first to take you to the appropriate subdirectory and then to 'fire up' the program:

   cd\WORDPR
   WP

With the PATH command, all you do is type the following:

   c:WP

The PATH command helps the computer to find the right subdirectory for you. You only have to type in the letters that start up your wordprocessor (or database, or spreadsheet). Whenever you add a subdirectory and a program to your hard disk, it is useful to make an appropriate addition to your PATH command line in your AUTOEXEC.BAT file. This can be done in any text editor but not, automatically, in any word-

What is 'housekeeping'?

processor. For more details about how to change your AUTOEXEC.BAT and CONFIG.SYS files, consult your DOS manual (see also the comments below). Figure 4.2 offers examples of the contents of simple AUTOEXEC.BAT and CONFIG.SYS files.

Naming subdirectories is rather like naming files; you can use up to eight letters to name a subdirectory although you cannot include an extension.

I find it useful to name subdirectories and files with names that are easily recognizable. For example, the subdirectory that contains the chapters of this book is called COMPUTE. Within that subdirectory, I have named the chapter files as follows:

```
C:\COMPUTE
  INTRO
  HEALTH.1
  TYPES.2
  BUYING.3
  HOUSEK.4
  WORDPR.5
  DATAB.6
  OTHER.7
  SHAREW.8
  WRITEG.9
  RESEARCH.10
  APPENDIX.1
  APPENDIX.2
  BIBLIOG
```

In this way I can see at a glance both the number of the chapter (the extension) and what the chapter is about.

It is important to note that three files must be in your root directory: these are:

- COMMAND.COM which contains essential instructions for running DOS;
- CONFIG.SYS which configures your computer every time you start it up;
- AUTOEXEC.BAT which automatically starts up certain functions.

Although this is not absolutely essential for the running of your computer, it makes life so much easier that it might as well be.

There will also be two 'hidden' files in your root directory which are necessary for the running of your computer. It is vital that none of these files is deleted at any time. Some users prefer to keep the AUTOEXEC.BAT and the CONFIG.SYS file in their DOS directory. If you decide to do that, you must know how to adjust your CONFIG.SYS file so that it can 'tell' the computer where these files are. Learning how to make adjustments to the AUTOEXEC.BAT and CONFIG.SYS files is an important part of learning about the finer points of using personal computers. It is worth taking time to read more about these two files and about how they affect your machine. Whilst all DOS manuals cover these issues in some detail, they are not always very easy to read and to follow. A book that does make the whole subject very clear is *PC World DOS 5 Complete Handbook* which is reviewed at the end of this chapter.

Back-ups

It cannot be emphasized too much that you must back up any files that you store on your hard disk. Every time you write a new data file – a report, a chapter of a book, an article and so on – you must make sure that it is not only stored on your hard disk but also that it is copied to a floppy. You may want to get into the habit of backing up all of your work before you switch off the computer at the end of a session. Alternatively, you may want to 'back up as you go' and make copies as soon as you have written your file to disk.

If you have large amounts of data on a hard disk, you can use a back-up program which will help you by reading the files on your disk and only backing up new files or files that have been added to during the course of a session. Also, you may want to consider a large scale back-up device such as a tape streamer. A tape streamer backs up large amounts of data to a tape which is similar to an ordinary cassette tape. Again, programs are available for use with tape streamers which allow you to do selective back-ups.

You need not back up everything that is on your hard disk. If you have problems with a program, for example, you will always have the original program disks and you can reinstall the program if necessary. You always need to back up files that you make yourself. The overriding principle should be that your back-up procedure allows you, at any time, to reproduce everything that is currently on your hard disk. If you have files on your hard disk that you cannot afford to loose, back them up now.

You should also keep an 'emergency' disk. If your hard disk fails for any reason, you need to know that you can restart your computer from your floppy disk drive. In order to do this, prepare a disk that you do not use for anything else by using the command: FORMAT A: /s. The /s at the end of the command is known as a 'switch' and it tells DOS to write essential start-up files to your new disk. You can then use that disk to restart the computer if anything happens to your hard disk. You may also want to include the CONFIG.SYS and AUTOEXEC.BAT files on that disk. These will enable you to start your computer so that it exactly mimics a start-up from the hard disk. You place the disk in drive A or B and reboot your machine. Instead of trying to boot from the hard disk, the computer will automatically read the floppy disk in the disk drive and start up your computer from there.

Viruses

A computer virus is a self-contained piece of code whose aim is to replicate, preferably undetected. Computer viruses, self-evidently, are nothing to do with the medical world but can cause havoc in a computer. They are designed by people who want to disrupt computer systems and are transmitted by being put onto disks which are then circulated via the normal channels. Some viruses are of a 'slow release' sort. They sit in a data file until a certain date and then are triggered by the computer's internal clock. Some viruses are relatively harmless and simply cause a message to appear on the monitor screen. Others are not so benign and destroy data on hard disks. There is a number of ways in which you can protect yourself from virus infection but it has to be said that none of these is 100% effective: everyone who uses a computer runs some risk of their computer being invaded. Whilst it goes without saying that computer viruses have nothing to do with their biological counterparts, it is intriguing to note the ways in which many computer magazines cash in on the health care metaphor!

- Check all new program disks with a commercial virus checking program. If you use such a program, make sure that you get copies of all update disks that the company supplies.

- Do not copy files from other people's computers.
- Do not leave your computer on, at work, unattended.
- Don't allow other people to use your machine for inspecting the contents of disks or for running new programs.
- Look out for anything suspicious happening on your PC. Unexpected disk activity, a slowing down of your computer's performance or unexpected messages on the screen can all be symptomatic of virus infection.
- Make sure that any new computer you buy is thoroughly checked for viruses.
- Make sure that you perform regular back-ups of your hard disk. If your computer does become infected with a virus, you need to know that you can reinstall everything that is on your hard disk. However, if you discover that you do have a virus on your hard disk, do **not** back it up. In this case, the virus would also be backed up onto your floppies. Then, when you reinstalled the data from your floppies, you would also reintroduce your virus. Instead, use a program to get rid of the virus and then back up the whole of the hard disk.

There are a number of commercial software packages available that check for and deal with personal computer viruses. Most of them are updated regularly, for the virus situation is changing almost daily. Here are some of the anti-virus programs to look out for:

- Dr Solomon's Anti-Virus Toolkit
- Bates' VIS Anti-Virus Utilities
- First Software F-Prot
- McAree Associates' Scanner
- Norton Anti-Virus
- Sophos Sweep and Vaccine.

Further information about virus infection is available from:

- Computing Crime Unit of the Metropolitan and City Police (071 230 1176/7). The unit provides a crime prevention service and can advise corporate users on all aspects of computer security. They can also assist and advise people who are victims of computer crime.

What is 'housekeeping'?

- National Computing Centre (061 228 6333). This organization advises computer users on all computer-related security matters, including computer viruses.

Computing Tip 9

Plan out your database program with a pen and pad

Before you use a new database program, draw out a plan on paper. This will allow you to experiment in a way that you are not likely to find so easy when working on the screen.

Example software: **Norton Utilities (Symatec)**

Norton Utilities is a huge package of programs which every serious computer user will find helpful. The situation above is just one in which Utilities could help. It can rescue deleted files and even deleted disks.

Norton Utilities has been around, in various versions, for some years. This latest version offers a highly integrated but easy to use set of utility programs for anyone who wants to use and maintain his or her computer to the utmost. The various elements of the program are drawn together via a menu screen which can be operated either with a mouse or with the keyboard. It is intuitive to use and the program is simple to install. Indeed, the menu system is almost too easy to use. Norton Utilities contains some very powerful and (to the novice) potentially dangerous programs. It would not be difficult to find yourself firing up these parts of the programs. So key with care. Some parts of the program are not for the novice.

Here are some of the things that the Norton Utilities can do. First, as noted above, it can recover accidentally wiped data. It can also help in those cases where the computer crashes in the middle of a program leaving data scattered around your hard disk. It can also repair damaged data files and this function might be vital if you keep large database or spreadsheet files.

It can also speed up your hard disk. Over a period of time, the hard disk gets to be 'fragmented'. This means that bits of files are written all over it, in no particular order. Part of the Norton Utilities suite can rearrange your files 'end to end' or contiguously. This can speed up the functioning of your hard disk quite considerably. As if that were not enough, the Norton Utilities also offers you a disk cache, which stores frequently read data from your hard disk and acts as an extremely fast section of memory.

Norton Utilities might have been made for the compulsive 'fiddler'. It has so many functions – most of which seem interesting – that you can spend hours fine tuning your computer. I suspect that a whole generation of computer users is evolving, who produce very little from their machines but who always have those machines functioning optimally. As one example of the sort of thing that will appeal to fiddlers, on a colour screen, the program allows you to alter the basic screen colour and then the colour of the text that you type onto the screen.

As with most utility programs, Norton Utilities offers an extensive menuing and file management program. It allows you to bypass the DOS prompt and view all of your files in their directories and subdirectories. It also enables you to keep a list of your programs and start them up at the touch of a button. It also has an extensive 'help' section which is easy to use and genuinely helpful. It also has some of the best documentation I have read.

The Norton Utilities will quickly become an indispensable program for any health care professional who uses computers. If you do research, write essays or papers or store records and data, you will find everything in this batch of programs to enable you to work more effectively. The Norton Utilities is like a good insurance policy. Most of the time, you will not use it but when you do, you want to know that it works and that it can do what it says it can. The Norton Utilities suite does what it says it can and is likely to save your sanity in the long term.

Computing Tip 10

Do not have fields that are too large in your database programs

When you design a database, it is tempting to make the fields for data entry as large as possible, 'just in case' you need to enter long strings of information. Large fields – even empty ones – take up a lot of disk space and slow up the database program. Instead, work out fairly carefully how much space you really need.

FURTHER READING

MS-DOS Quick Reference (1991) Que Corporation, Carmel, Indiana

This slim volume puts most of the essential commands of MS-DOS at your fingertips. As is the case with many software manuals, the standard MS-DOS handbook does not make light reading. You often have to search through it to find the one command that you need. This quick reference book (one of a series that Que Corporation publishes) offers the various commands and utilities of MS-DOS listed in dictionary format. It is also a vital resource for DOS error messages, the DOS text editor and the making of batch files and using keyboard shortcuts. This is the sort of book that you want to keep next to your keyboard.

Socha, J. and Hicks, C. (1991) *PC World DOS 5 Complete Handbook*, IDG Books, distributed by Computer Manuals, 50 James Road, Tyseley, Birmingham B11 2BA

The first part of this exhaustive manual takes an unusual approach to teaching you all about DOS. It comes complete with a special edition of the program Norton Commander. The early chapters show you how to use this to get the best out of DOS. Following chapters take a more conventional approach to all aspects of the DOS operating system. The second half of the book is an alphabetical listing and discussion of all the DOS commands. It is much more detailed than the DOS manual and offers interesting tricks and tips that the authors have learned over the years. If you only want to buy one book about DOS, then this is probably the one. It is detailed, helpful and written in a clear and sometimes personal style.

Oberlin, S., Kervran, P. and Cox, J. (1992) *A Quick Course in Windows 3.1*, Online Press Books, distributed by Computer Manuals, 50 James Road, Tyseley, Birmingham B11 2BA

This is a straightforward and useful guide to using all aspects of Windows. The book is large format but it is designed to lay flat when opened. It can easily be propped up in front of your computer as you work through it. Considerable thought has gone into the layout and pacing of this book. The authors explain everything in a simple and readable way and define terms as they go. The book is illustrated with clear screen shots so that you can easily check what should be on the screen at any given time. This is the ideal book for anyone who is starting out with Windows and can't face one of the bigger manuals. In particular, the book helps you to:

- organize your programs and files logically;
- work with several programs at the same time;
- transfer information between files without quitting and restarting programs;
- work with both Windows and non-Windows applications;
- use Notepad, Calendar, CardFile, Calculator, Terminal, Recorder and all the other tools that are included with the Windows program.

5 Wordprocessing

The wordprocessor is the most frequently used of all computer programs. Any health professional who uses a computer at home or at work is likely to need to get to grips with one sooner or later. Most people, once they get the hang of them, wonder how they managed without. This chapter is about all aspects of wordprocessing as it applies to health professionals.

WHAT IS WORDPROCESSING?

Wordprocessing means never having to rewrite from scratch. Essentially, you type your text into the computer, in any form you like. You can write full sentences, notes, paragraphs that follow logically and those that don't. Afterwards, you can go back and make substantial changes to what you have written. For example, you can:

- move the text around;
- delete words, sentences and whole blocks of words;
- spellcheck your work;
- change the margin size around your text . . . and so on.

Working with a wordprocessor is similar to typing but allows you to do far more. One important point needs to be made right from the start: there is no need to do a 'carriage return' at the end of each line. As the text you type fills up the screen, the computer program 'word wraps' the text so that it can flow over onto the next line.

Learn how a wordprocessor functions. Learn about the things that it can do automatically and about the things that you need to do yourself. If you have never used one before, you may be pleasantly surprised how much automation can be used and how useful it can be. If you have used a wordprocessor before, fiddle with some of the functions you haven't used so far. Again, you will probably be surprised at the things that you have missed.

One final word in this section: learn to type. I am often surprised at the number of people who use very fast and very sophisticated wordprocessors but slow down the whole process of working because they have to hover, with two fingers, over the keys. Touch-typing can help you to make full use of your wordprocessor.

USES IN HEALTH CARE SETTINGS

Wordprocessors have taken over from typewriters in most settings. Here are some of the uses to which they can be put in the health care field:

- preparation of essays, projects and reports;
- development of hand-outs and other educational tools;
- preparation of questionnaires and other research instruments;
- analysis of qualitative data;
- recording of notes about patients and clients;
- writing of articles, journal papers and books;
- writing of day-to-day correspondence and memos.

Think about the amount of writing that you do in your job. Then decide whether or not the writing tasks that you are engaged in could be made easier with some automation. Usually, they could.

VARIETIES OF WORDPROCESSOR

There are various ways of dividing up the types of wordprocessors that are available. Figure 5.1 illustrates some of the different sorts. As ever, it is important to try out a number of different programs, if you can, before you decide which is the best one for you. Wordprocessors, for some

DOS-based wordprocessors e.g. WordPerfect, WordStar, Word	Windows-based wordprocessors e.g. WordPerfect for Windows, WordStar for Windows, Word for Windows
Shareware wordprocessors e.g. Galaxy, PC-Write	Commercial wordprocessors e.g. WordPerfect, Word
Low price wordprocessors e.g. LocoScript PC, TopCopy	Full price wordprocessors e.g. WordPerfect, WordStar
Fully featured wordprocessors e.g. Word, WordPerfect	Less fully featured wordprocessors e.g. Format-PC, Tassword

Figure 5.1 Different types of wordprocessors.

reason, generate disciples. Some people believe that the wordprocessor that they use is, necessarily, the only one to use! Beware of evangelists!

There is usually a relation between price and functionality. Fully featured wordprocessors that have very sophisticated features tend to cost more. It does not always follow, though, that fully featured wordprocessors are more complicated to use. Some have a 'simple' version of the program that can be employed until the user wants to try some of the more complicated features. Most wordprocessors now offer a range of ways of working. Many use a series of 'pull-down' menus, from which the user selects a particular function. Many, too, make full use of 'macros' or short-cut keystroke combinations.

CHECKLIST OF WORDPROCESSING FUNCTIONS

Not all wordprocessors offer the same range of features although most of the larger ones are comparable. The following is a list of functions to consider before you buy or change your wordprocessor. Not everyone needs one that does everything. On the other hand, it is surprising what you find yourself using if you have the facilities!

- **Cut.** This is a fundamental wordprocessing feature. The ability to cut blocks of text, sentences or paragraphs from your document is essential.

Computing Tip 11	**Clean out your hard disk regularly**
	It is surprising easy to collect files on your hard disks – files that you do not need. You may, for example, have programs that make temporary files which are not automatically erased when you leave the program. Unwanted files can clog up your hard disk and make it run more slowly. Also, unwanted files take up space that could be used for important files. Every month, comb through the files on your hard disk and carefully erase the ones that you do not need. Try to keep the root directory empty of files other than COMMAND.COM, AUTOEXEC.BAT and CONFIG.SYS. On the other hand, erase files from the root directory with extreme care: it is vital that you do **not** erase these three files!

- **Paste.** Another important feature. Most wordprocessors allow you to copy or move text from one part of a document to another. When you move text in this way, it is known as 'cutting and pasting' – a hangover, presumably, from the printing trade.
- **Search and replace.** Most wordprocessors with allow you to automatically search for a particular word or phrase in a document. Most will also let you automatically replace it with a different word or phrase. Imagine, for example, that you had prepared a report in which Mrs Jones, a social worker, featured often. Imagine, then, that the social worker left your organization and was replaced by a Dr Black. With the search and replace feature, you could quickly change all references to 'Mrs Jones' to 'Dr Black'. You can use the search and replace feature to remove a particular word or phrase throughout a document. In this case, you simply invoke the search and replace feature, ask it to search for the word or phrase and leave the replace feature blank.

    The search feature can also be used simply to find a particular word or phrase. Instead of searching visually through a document for a particular word or heading, you let the search feature do the work for you.
- **Spellchecker.** If your spelling is anything like mine, this is also an essential feature. More sophisticated wordprocessors will also flag

up double words ('She left left the clinic later that afternoon') and allow you to add your own words to the spellchecking 'dictionary'. Be careful when you do this. It is quite easy to add incorrect spellings to a spellchecker, out of ignorance! Once you have done this, your spellchecker will no longer try to correct your mistake.

- **Word counter.** If you are preparing a research report or a thesis that has to be of a particular length or less than a given number of words, then you need a word counting function. In some wordprocessors, you can only get a word count after you have run the spellchecking function, which can be frustrating.

- **Footnote and/or endnote generator.** Some of the top-end wordprocessors offer you the ability to automatically generate footnotes and/or endnotes. If you later add more foot or endnotes, the number of the previous ones is automatically adjusted. This is a particularly powerful function but one to use cautiously. Footnotes, in particular, are generally felt to be more annoying than useful. If you are thinking of using them, try to write what you have to say into the main body of the text. This is one area in which computing has helped writers a great deal. Presumably, in the past, footnotes were widely used because authors and researchers did not want to rewrite large sections of their work in order to incorporate new ideas. Instead, they added footnotes. Wordprocessing has made it easy to change what you have written. Today, there should be no need to use footnotes or endnotes.

- **Auto back-up facilities.** It is important that you back up what you write in your wordprocessor as you write it. Thus, when you pause, it is helpful if you are able to press a key and what you have written is backed up to the hard disk. Better still is if the program automatically backs up what you have written. One wordprocessor – Topcopy Professional – automatically writes both to screen and to disk at the same time, but this is rare. Other programs allow you to adjust the time delay between writes to disk. I have found it useful to set my wordprocessor to back up what is on the screen every five minutes. It should be noted, however, that this writing to disk does not remove the necessity of backing up all of your new work to floppy disks at the end of your wordprocessing session.

- **Zoom features.** If your wordprocessor is not one that works directly in Windows mode, what you see on the screen will not match, exactly, what you see on the printed page. Many wordprocessors, however, have a zoom feature which allows you to see what a printed page will look like, before you print it out. You may also be allowed to zoom in on one section of the page, by enlarging the image on the screen.

- **Import facilities.** You need to be sure that the wordprocessor you choose can import files from other programs if this is going to be important to you. You may, for example, want to import data from your database into your wordprocessor. It is essential that you check, before buying, that this can be done.

- **Export facilities.** This is the reverse of the above issue. You may want to export material that you have written in your wordprocessor into your database, spreadsheet, graphics or desktop publishing program. Again, you need to know, before you buy, whether or not this can be done. It is usually possible to use a 'universal' format, called ASCII, for importing or exporting data.

- **File manager.** You need to be able to view and manage the files that you produce. Nearly all wordprocessors have file managers that allow you to call up, save, delete and copy files that you have produced. Some are easier to use than others.

- **Windows compatibility.** Whilst you can run most wordprocessors under Windows, there are some that are written specifically for Windows and which make full use of the graphical user interface elements of that program. You need to know, in advance, whether or not your program is a 'Windows compatible' or a 'Windows only' product.

- **Thesaurus.** A thesaurus is one method of finding synonyms. A number of the larger wordprocessing programs include an on-line thesaurus.

- **Grammar checker.** Many wordprocessors now include a grammar checker which will give you a detailed analysis of your writing in terms of its grammar and readability. This may be useful if you are trying to write for a particular audience or a specific journal.

- **Graphics editor.** Many wordprocessors now include many desktop publishing features. The ability to include graphics (pictures, diagrams, graphs, etc.) may be important to you.

Checklist of wordprocessing functions 83

- **Equation editor.** If you work with mathematical data, you may need a wordprocessor that can write and edit equations.
- **Table editor.** Many types of writing in the health professions call for the use of tables and charts. A table editor will help you to produce boxed diagrams. Some are superb.
- **Styles feature.** A styles editor allows you to set up certain predetermined layouts. You may, for example, want a consistent layout for one particular project and another, but different, for a report you are writing. In this case, with a style feature, you could develop two different styles, each of which could be quickly called up to shape the structure of your document.
- **Macros feature.** Macros are collections of keypresses that can be played out by pressing just one key. You may, for example, want to set up a macro that will automatically double space the document you have written, change the margin sizes and count the words in it. Macros can save you a lot of time if you often use a variety of functions in your wordprocessors. With some wordprocessors, you can customize your keyboard in almost infinitely variable ways – even to the point of redesignating the functions of the letter keys! If you don't like the normal QWERTY layout, you can change it. I don't advise it, though.
- **Centre text.** Most wordprocessors allow you to automatically centre single lines or blocks of text.
- **Date feature.** Some programs will let you enter the date into a document at the press of a key. Some will also automatically 'update' the function. If, for example, you type a letter on 15.4.93 but do not print it out until 30.5.93, the wordprocessor will automatically update the letter for you. This is particularly useful if you use 'standard' letters that you send out on different dates.
- **Multiple screens.** Sometimes, you need to work on more than one document at any one time. You may, for example, want to cut and paste text between two or more documents. Wordprocessors that enable you to view multiple screens of text allow you to work in this way.
- **Printer drivers.** Make sure that your wordprocessor will be able to send your documents to your printer. Do not assume that every wordprocessor can automatically recognize any given printer.

- **Underlining, italicizing and emboldening.** Almost all wordprocessors allow you to italicize or embolden words, sentences or blocks of text. As a rule, use these functions sparingly.

- **Mail merging.** Mail merging is the process by which you can develop a standard letter and then have your wordprocessor prepare multiple copies, all of which have appropriate names and addresses on them. If you have ever received junk mail which looks as though it is addressed to you personally, then you have seen the outcome of mail merging. It can be useful to health care professionals who need to write the same sort of letter to many clients and to the researcher who wants to 'personalize' a questionnaire.

- **Outlining.** All American students are taught to outline before writing essays. An outlining funtion allows you to 'play' with headings and subheadings before deciding the order of a piece of prose or a report. A useful tool for making your work more structured.

- **Context-sensitive help.** Sometimes you need help when you are working with your wordprocessor. Almost all programs enable you to call up help screens – usually (but not always) by pressing the F1 function key. Context-sensitive help is an advanced sort of help. Imagine, for example, that you are trying to add words to your spellchecker. You get to a menu that you think is the one that will enable you to do this . . . but you are not sure. Pressing the appropriate help key when context-sensitive help is present will take you straight to a help screen that is about the spellchecker. In other words, wherever you are in the program, help for that part of the program is always to hand. This is particularly useful when you are learning to use a wordprocessor for the first time.

- **Mouse support.** Many, but not all, wordprocessors allow you to use a mouse for certain functions. Typically, a mouse may be used to 'block' text for copying or moving. Sometimes, too, the mouse can be used to make choices from menu screens. Not everyone likes using a mouse and some are irritated at having to take their hands off the keyboard. On the other hand, if you use a Windows specific wordprocessor, the mouse will usually be an essential part of the program's operation. Decide, before you choose your wordprocessor, whether or not you see yourself as a mouse fan.

- **Page layout.** Most wordprocessors will allow you to set automatic page numbering. Some will let you reset that numbering to run from a certain page. Imagine, for example, that you were writing a report and 'page 1' was to be the first page of Chapter 1 of that report and not the 'actual' first page of the document. Certain wordprocessors can enable you to arrange this – and even to use Roman numerals for the preceding pages.

The page layout functions of some computers will include such esoteric items such as 'kerning': automatic control over the distance between certain letters and numbers when a document is printed out. If you look at the following phrase: 'We would like to go to Watford', you will notice that, in a printed book, the gap between the 'W' and the 'e' of 'We' is smaller than the gap between the 'g' and the 'o' of 'go'. This is kerning. In a laser printed document, the difference that kerning can make can be important. Kerning makes no difference to documents printed on a dot matrix printer, which cannot support it.

Most wordprocessors will let you decide on whether you want a 'ragged right' margin or a 'justified right'. Laser printed documents usually look better with right justification and dot matrix ones better with ragged right. Here is an illustration of the difference between the two:

Justified right margin
This paragraph is an example of the use of a right justified margin setting. The net effect is that both margins are parallel and text is distributed evenly along the lines. Justified right text can sometimes be more difficult to read if printing quality is not particularly good. Traditionally, of course, typists could not produce documents which used justification in this way.

Ragged right margin
This paragraph is an example of the use of a ragged right margin. Some people find computer generated output that has a ragged right margin easier to read. Sometimes, journal editors prefer you to submit manuscripts which have ragged right margins. On the other hand, books are only very rarely printed in this way. Increasingly, justified right margins are becoming the norm.

You may, if you wish, centre text and even right justify it, with a ragged left. Here are examples of the use of centring and right justification:

This is centred text
It is best reserved for major headings
You may want to use it for the title of an essay, project or report

This is an example of a passage that is justified on the right and ragged on the left. It should be used very sparingly (if at all). It can sometimes be used with good effect in short passages of text in a 'desktop published' document. Magazines sometimes use it to highlight small portions of text.

Computing Tip 12

Defragment the hard disk regularly

As a hard disk fills up, the files on it get split up and data is written to different parts of the disk. This data is then accessed much more slowly by your programs. Use a defragmenting program (they are available with both PC-TOOLS and Norton Utilities) once a month to make sure that all your data is written contiguously.

COLLECTIVE WRITING

One of the possibilities that wordprocessing opens up is that of a group of people writing together. Many health professionals – especially those who work in the academic world – want or need to publish but do not necessarily want to write on their own. The wordprocessor enables one person to write notes or rough paragraphs, another to add to those drafts and yet a third to edit. This way of working is ideal when it comes to editing books, papers and projects. Monteith (1992) takes this idea further when she suggests that students can also work in this way:

> The likelihood of actual collaborative writing becomes more possible, beyond any basic advice with editing and redrafting. At the less contentious level, for instance, students can help each other with their writing. In my second-year class one student was having trouble writing the end of her documentary. She typed in the version she

had written which was networked to other computers. This procedure could also have been accomplished with disks and stand-alone computers. Other students reworked her version as they saw fit. The student then took away eight other versions of the ending, which she said proved very helpful.

Monteith covers many of the possibilities of collaborative wordprocessing. First, she suggests that such writing can be done via a network of computers. If such a bank of computers is networked in a health care setting, it means that many professionals can work on a range of documents together. This opens up the possibility of speedily producing research reports, papers for publication and discussion papers. Second, she points out that the same method of working can be achieved with stand-alone computers by simply swapping disks. Again, in a health care setting, this might mean that one colleague works on a paper at home, swaps disks with another colleague who takes that disk home and edits it. I have worked with a colleague in this way when editing a book. As chapter authors submitted their manuscripts (on disk), we took turns in taking each one home to work on. Then, we swapped disks and reviewed each other's work. This did at least two things. It allowed for more detailed editing and checking. It also encouraged us to pay attention to continuity of style. As we were both working on the same manuscripts, in the same medium but on different nights, we were soon able to establish a 'rhythm' of writing.

Perhaps the most contentious of Monteith's points is whether or not students should be allowed to work in this way towards papers for assessment. If we consider the situation before wordprocessing, it is doubtful that we would have encouraged students to write sections of each other's essays. The 'anonymity' of wordprocessing seems to have broken this taboo. It remains an open question as to whether or not all academics in all health care settings will accept this way of working.

Example software: **WordPerfect (WordPerfect UK)**

WordPerfect is the world leader in the wordprocessing field. It is available in both DOS and Windows versions and the Windows version is discussed below. The program offers almost every function you could want and its functions can be invoked in a number of ways. First, you can use the 'function' keys along the top of the keyboard to trigger the various functions directly. If you prefer, you can work with sets of menus that can be dropped down from the top of the screen. You can also work with a mouse and avoid keystrokes altogether. You can 'personalize' the program by completely rewriting the keyboard to suit your own preferences. This, combined with the ability to create 'macros' – shortcut keystrokes that invoke the functions of your choice – go to make WordPerfect one of the most versatile wordprocessors on the market.

Like all wordprocessors, WordPerfect can manipulate text in a variety of ways. You can cut and paste blocks of words, spellcheck what you have written and you can count the number of words in a document. You can embolden and italicize at the touch of a button, number pages and put your words into columns if you so choose. There is also an on-board thesaurus for checking for synonyms. Most printers are supported by the program and WordPerfect always responds quickly to requests for new printer drivers.

WordPerfect overlaps with some desktop publishing programs. You can draw boxes and diagrams with it and import graphics into your work. You can also check to see what your completed work looks like in its printed format through the program's 'view document' function which can show you the whole of an A4 page at a time. This is handy when you have finished writing and want to check your paragraph and margin settings.

For larger documents such as dissertations, theses and book manuscripts, the program has a useful master document function. This allows you to work on single chapters of a manuscript and then to bring all those chapters together into a large, single document for editing, page numbering, spellchecking and so forth. Once you have done these things, you can then divide your manuscript back into its component parts. The program also has full mail merging facilities and the ability to create footnotes, endnotes, contents pages and indexes. You can also work in two documents concurrently which is particularly useful if you want to refer to notes. The outlining feature is also helpful in structuring your work.

WordPerfect has a refreshing policy on use of the program. A single copy that is installed on a single computer at work can be copied on to one person's computer at home. Thus, two working copies can be available to the user as long as there is no possibility of their being used at the same time. This also means that if you use the program at work, you could also use the same copy on a notebook computer when you travel.

Example software: **WordPerfect for Windows (WordPerfect UK)**

This is the Windows version of the product described above. To run it, users will need a fast computer with at least 2Mb of RAM and a fairly large hard disk. The program will run much more quickly with 4Mb or more of memory.

The program is simple to load and easy to start from the Windows environment. It does, however, take a while to load and this time factor is highlighted throughout the product. It is slow to scroll through documents but much more so when it is processing commands.

The graphic interface is good. The user is presented with a clear screen and a 'what you see is what you get' format for text, boxes and graphics. As always with a WordPerfect product, the program can be easily tailored to your own requirements. Working with this sort of program grows on you. If you are familiar with WordPerfect, you will quickly get the hang of WordPerfect for Windows. Once familiar, it seems likely that most will want to stay with the new format.

The 'button bar' is a particularly useful function. The user can define his or her own set of 'push buttons' at the bottom or side of the screen and these are 'pressed' with the mouse. Buttons can trigger wordprocessing functions or can be linked to macros. I found it useful to design buttons that triggered the word counting and spelling functions and later I can envisage developing a wide range of 'linked' buttons that will allow me to do almost anything in the program without reference to the menu system. This makes the program both time saving and easy to use.

The regular WordPerfect user can have the program running in a format in which most of the original key combinations are retained. This may be the key to WordPerfect for Windows' success.

WordPerfect for Windows is likely to appeal to the many health care professionals who already use WordPerfect. If you want to switch to a Windows environment, this is the wordprocessor to go for. Writers, researchers and program planners in all parts of the health care professions will find this a valuable and useful product.

> **Computing Tip 13**
>
> **Take frequent breaks**
>
> Computers can be seductive. If you are not careful, you can sit at one for hours. This is not particularly good for your posture, nor for your hands and wrists. Take frequent breaks. Get up and make yourself a cup of coffee, or get some exercise, at least once an hour. During such breaks you can set your computer to count words or create an index – tasks that normally take a few minutes on longer documents.

Example software: **LetterPerfect (WordPerfect UK)**

LetterPerfect is the ideal small to middle-sized wordprocessor. Easy to install, simple to work with and comprehensive in features, it is an excellent program for those who are new to computers and wordprocessors. It will also be ideal for computers with limited memory or for the smaller notebook or laptop computers.

LetterPerfect is supplied on both 3½" and 5¼" disks and installs itself. The initial editing screen is bare except for a small line at the bottom of the screen which tells you what page you are working on. The program's functions can be called up from a set of pull-down menus or by the use of the function keys that run along the top of the computer keyboard. WordPerfect has come in for a lot of criticism for the apparent arbitrariness of the allocation of functions to these keys. The company does, however, supply a cardboard strip that you can sit just above the function keys. In fact a whole number of these strips is supplied so that you can find the perfect match with your computer. These strips tell you what each of the keys does and it doesn't take long to work out the 'logic' of the allocation of keys.

LetterPerfect is not only simple to use, it is also very fast. Whilst there is never very much to see on the screen, help is always available at the press of the F3 function key. Help is context-sensitive and so you can always find out what to do next if you get stuck. It also interfaces well with other WordPerfect programs and will accept and edit WordPerfect files.

The program also comes with the company's menuing system, WordPerfect Shell. This allows you to set up a user-friendly menu when you first turn on the computer. You can adjust Shell so that each of your programs (including LetterPerfect) is allocated a letter. When you press that letter on the keyboard, your program starts up. A more detailed version of Shell is also available as a separate program, when it is known as WordPerfect Office (see pp. 55–7). The inclusion of Shell makes this wordprocessor even better value. It also enables you to transfer data between LetterPerfect and other programs.

SETTING UP YOUR WORDPROCESSOR

Wordprocessors are all supplied, preset, with certain basic settings. These are known as 'defaults'. An example of a default setting is that most wordprocessors will be set to have margin settings of 1" all round the page. All such settings can be modified to suit the way that you work. As you get to know more about the wordprocessor of your choice, experiment with the default settings and, as necessary, change or modify them. Do not take it for granted that the default settings are necessarily the best settings.

Examples of defaults that you can reset and have running with new definitions include the following:

- **Colours.** You can usually change both the background and the foreground settings of your computer screen, if you are working with a colour monitor. You may find that a blue background with yellow or white letters or graphics is a workable combination. It is best not to be too extravagant with your colour settings if you plan to sit at your computer for prolonged periods.

- **Back-up settings.** Modern wordprocessors automatically back up the file that you are working on to the hard disk, at preset intervals. You can set the time limit for this. You must still make regular back-ups of your hard disk files to floppies.

- **Column and/or table settings.** Not all wordprocessors allow you to use columns and tables, but many do. You can modify the format of these as you work so that they are as large or as small as you need.
- **Font sizes.** A font is a style or a 'family' of print-faces. This book, for example, is printed in a font called Palatino. Most wordprocessors allow you to work in different-sized letters and numbers. With some, you may see the difference on the screen. With others, the changes in font size will only show up when you print out a document. Many wordprocessors have a 'preview' function that allows you to see what a printed document will look like before you print it out.
- **Headers and footers** can be produced 'automatically' by many wordprocessors. Use these sparingly. Although printed books and magazines have running headers and footers it is not a good idea to use them in manuscripts that you send to editors of magazines, journals or books. They only have to cross them through when they are editing your work.
- **Justification.** You may prefer to have both margins flush or to have the words at the right margin 'ragged'. Generally speaking, laser printed pages look better with justification turned on, whilst dot matrix printed pages look better with it turned off ('ragged right').
- **Keyboard layout.** Some wordprocessors allow you to modify your keyboard considerably. You may, for example, want to change the function of some of the keys that you rarely or never use. You can allocate such keys to perform macro functions – shortcut keystrokes that allow you to get your wordprocessor to perform complicated functions quickly. For example, on my keyboard, I have set up the '*' key (on the right hand side of the keyboard), which I never otherwise use, to print 'bullets' to the screen for use in lists such as this one. Producing 'bullets' is normally quite a complicated procedure but a macro speeds up the process.
- **Line spacing.** Double line spacing is often a requirement for manuscripts that are submitted to editors for publication. Most wordprocessors allow you considerable latitude in the setting of line spacing.
- **Page numbering.** Almost all wordprocessors allow you to set automatic page numbering. Many also allow you to decide where you show the page numbers on the printed page. I always set this to 'bottom, middle' but this is as much a matter of taste as anything.

- **Paper and page size.** Although paper comes in various sizes, there is only one paper size for writing: A4. Do not use smaller or larger sizes. Also, buy fairly good paper of about 80 gsm in weight. For posting work to publishers or to magazines and journals, do not use heavier paper than this otherwise your bill for stamps will be rather large. Use plain paper and not 'laid'. Laid paper has faint lines running through it in the style of a watermark. Do not, as a rule, use coloured paper of any sort for documents.
- **Right and left margins.** The margin settings on all wordprocessors can be changed to suit the way that you work and to suit the final layout of the printed page. I tend to have my margins set at 1½″ all round. In this way, I can always see the whole of a line of text across the screen. Narrow margin settings usually mean that the text disappears off the edge of the monitor screen as you are typing down the page. Remember, too, that it is possible to have one type of margin setting for use while working at the screen and another for printing out documents.
- **Tab settings.** The usual default for tab settings is about an inch. This setting is quite useful for producing indentations at the beginnings of paragraphs although you are free to set the tabs at lesser or greater settings.
- **Top and bottom margins.** Allow fairly generous margins at the top and bottom of documents. Small top and bottom margins tend to make wordprocessed documents look cramped. I have mine set to 1½″ for top, bottom and sides.
- **Underlining style.** You can usually set up your wordprocessor to underline words and spaces or just words. It is usual to underline both words and spaces. If you are printing out on a laser printer, you may prefer to use italics rather than underlining in your work. In a manuscript, underlining is used to represent passages that will be printed as italics in the final publication.

FURTHER READING

Rimmer, S. (1991) *The Home Office Computer Book*, Sybex Inc., distributed by Computer Manuals, 50 James Road, Tyseley, Birmingham B11 2BA

A book with this title would seem to be about the ins and outs of working from home. The introduction is about this. It discusses the fact that many people are now using computers as part of a home office. After that, the book is all about computing in general. No further reference is made, specifically, to home office working. It is, however, an extremely well written and detailed book for anyone who wants to become more familiar with the process of computing. It is written by a computer journalist of many years' experience and this experience shows. Authors are often anonymous but in this book, the author is never far away and his personal ideas are both helpful and entertaining. The book is not only informative but it is also easy and interesting to read. It discusses the use of both IBM and compatible computers and Apple Macintoshes. It is rare to find a book which offers fairly objective advice about the pros and cons of both approaches to computing. It also helps you to decide which the best system might be for you to use at home.

The first chapter is a straightforward discussion of what computers are, the different types and how to choose one. The next two chapters discuss printers and operating systems. Again, the style is clear and straightforward. Operating systems, in particular, are often difficult to describe in writing and the author is to be congratulated on his ability to convey the basics of DOS and Windows in such a straightforward way.

Later chapters cover the basics of wordprocessing, desktop publishing, graphics, databases and spreadsheets. There are also chapters on setting up a modem and using faxes. All of these chapters review a range of hard and software and all offer the author's own experience of working with a range of products. Anyone reading these chapters should be much clearer about what to look for in the very crowded (and often expensive) market place.

The book closes with interesting chapters on utility programs and shareware.

6 Databases

The term database has two sorts of meanings. First, in computing, it refers to a program which helps to organize and structure data in such a way as to make it easily retrievable. Second, in a more general sense, it refers to a collection of data itself. In this chapter, both sorts of database are discussed. In the first half of the chapter, database programs are explored. In the second half, collections of data useful to health care professionals and stored on compact disks, are identified. The first half, then, is how you organize your own data. The second half is data that is already organized for you.

DATABASE PROGRAMS: ESSENTIALS

There are two main types of database programs: the fixed form database and the free form database. A fixed form database is rather like a card index system. It has labelled areas (known as 'fields') in which you enter your data. Each 'card' is known as a 'form'. Before you start using your database, you have to design your 'form' and make decisions about how many fields to have and how long each of the 'fields' should be. Figure 6.1 clarifies these points.

You can usually have a large number of fields in a form that you design for your database. Sometimes, though, the amount of data that you can enter into any given field is limited. Often, this limitation is as few as 250 characters. This means that you cannot simply type in page after page of data into the 'comments' section of the form illustrated in the figure above. To use pages of data rather than short words or sentences, you need a free form database.

A free form database does not work with the notions of forms and

---

This whole diagram represents a database 'form'. Each form has a number of fixed length 'fields'

Surname .... (this is one field)

First names .... (this is another field)

Address: ....
.... (this is a third, and longer field)

Comments ....
.... (this is a fourth field)

Figure 6.1 A form, containing fields, in a database.

fields. With a free form database, you simply type in your data and save it. When you want to find a particular piece of information, you simply conduct a 'search' for the particular data you want. Figure 6.2 illustrates one possible entry in a free form database. It illustrates some notes that a health care researcher may keep about a research project.

If the health professional who used this kind of free form database wanted to view this information on screen, all he or she would have to do is search on the words 'David', 'JP', 'introduction' or any other word that appears in the data. Clearly, other entries may also have these words and many free form databases allow you to search on more than one word, such as 'David and JP'. The free form database is a convenient way of storing types of data that do not fit into a regular structure.

CHOOSING A DATABASE

Here are some questions you may want to ask yourself before you decide on the database that will suit you best. Also bear in mind that people's tastes differ. Some like complicated and colourful programs that do almost everything. Others like simplicity. On the whole, it is probably better to plump for simplicity if you are not sure.

> David Jones: Interview Number 16
>
> I met David through an introduction from JP. He may be able to help with the project by acting as an interview respondent. He has had a number of admissions to hospital and many of them have been 'unpleasant'. He is articulate and seems eager to co-operate.
>
> Things to do:
>
> - Contact JP again and ask for David's address
> - Write to David and ask for an interview
> - Check his status before interviewing
>
> After this interview, check all others and cross reference as necessary.

Figure 6.2 Example of one entry in a free form database.

- What do I want to use the program for?
- Will I be printing from the database?
- Will I want to transfer entries from my database to my wordprocessor?
- Will I need to use a codeword to enter my database? This is particularly important if confidential information is to be stored.
- Do I need a fixed form or a free form database?
- Can I change the structure of the forms once I have entered data?
- How much is the program?
- Will other people be using it?
- Can I design my own screen formats for data entry?
- Can I get help, quickly, if I need to?
- Have I seen the program up and running?
- What books are available about the product?
- How many other people do I know who use this type of database?

> **Computing Tip 14**
>
> **Back up important data twice**
>
> ALWAYS back up your work to floppy disks. When your hard disk crashes (and it will, one day) you stand to lose all of your data if you do not have back-ups. For very important work, have a second set of back-up disks that you keep in another location. If, for example, you are writing a dissertation or thesis, keep two copies of your work on two sets of disks. Keep one of those sets at home and another at work. Then, in the unlikely event that your hard disk and your floppies don't work, you will always have another copy of your project. Everyone who works in colleges and universities can tell horror stories of students who did not have copies of their theses or dissertations and who subsequently and accidentally reformatted their hard disks!

USING DATABASES IN THE HEALTH CARE PROFESSIONS

There are numerous uses for computerized databases. Any information that falls into categories is likely to be usefully stored in this way and some unstructured material can be stored in a free form database. First some basic principles:

- Decide whether you will use a fixed form or a free form database system. Both have advantages and disadvantages. For very structured data, such as names and addresses and patient or client records, the fixed form database is probably best. If you plan to record notes and other loosely structured material, the freeform database may suit you best. All of the other principles below apply only to using the fixed form database. With the other sort, all you do is enter your data!

- Make sure that you are completely familiar with the program you plan to use. Explore features such as field size, number of available fields in any given form, printing features, report production and transfer of data into your wordprocessor.

- Plan out your database form on paper before you turn on the computer. Drawing out the form with a pen or pencil is much more likely to produce the overall plan that you need. You can cross out, modify field sizes and so forth in a way that may not be possible on the computer screen.

- Think very carefully about how to divide up your fields. In a name and address database, for example, you may or may not need to divide up the first names and the surname. You may or may not want to divide the address into separate fields for street, town, postcode and so on. If you think it likely that you will want to use just the town name on a particular occasion, or if you are likely to want to search for the town name, breaking down the address can be useful. On the other hand, the more fields you use, the more space you are likely to use on your hard disk. Also, with more fields, the database tends to slow up when you have to work with it. Have enough fields but do not have too many.

- Make sure that your database will allow you to change the format of your form once you have devised it and have begun to enter data. If you have planned your form well, on paper, you are unlikely to need to make changes. Often, though, it is not until you start to use the database 'for real' that you realize that you should have had one or two more fields. Some database programs do not let you make modifications to a form once you have entered data.

There are two other ways of dividing up database types. Fixed form databases can be either flat file or relational. Whilst the difference between these two types is worthy of a book on its own, they can be distinguished as follows. A flat file database is like a card file. You can open up the file and search through it for the entries that you want. With a flat file database, you can search just the data entries that are in a particular file. A relational database allows you to call up information from a number of files. Thus, you may keep the names and addresses of your students in one file and their exam results in another. With a relational database, you can do a quick search of names, addresses and marks, in one go. With a flat file database, you cannot. Generally speaking, relational databases are more powerful but take considerably more planning if they are to work successfully. If your needs are simple, then a flat file database is likely to be sufficient. Most of the larger commercial programs that are available today are of the relational sort but all can also be used as flat file databases.

THE DATA PROTECTION ACT

Anyone who stores information about other people should be aware of their obligations under the Data Protection Act of 1984. The Act recognizes the special importance of personal data and the individual citizen's rights. These are expressed in the requirements of the Act, which are as follows:

- All computer bureaux must be registered; all personal data and intended uses for that data must be registered with the Data Protection Registrar and used solely in accordance with the declared objectives of registration. Data may not be sent abroad unless this is specifically permitted by the terms of registration. Individuals about whom data is held (data subjects) have a right to be informed about its nature and contents.
- Any person owning a computer used to process personal data (data user), must do so in accordance with the principles of the Act, namely:
- The personal data shall be processed fairly and lawfully.
- Personal data shall be held only for one or more specified and lawful purposes.
- Personal data held for any purpose must be adequate, relevant and not excessive in relation to that purpose or those purposes.
- Personal data shall be accurate and, where necessary, kept up-to-date.
- Personal data held for any purpose or purposes shall not be kept longer than is necessary for that purpose or purposes.

The Act also stipulates that an individual shall be entitled at reasonable intervals and without undue expense or delay:

- To be informed by any data user whether he or she holds any personal data of which that individual is the subject and to have access to any such data held by a data user and, where appropriate, to have such data corrected or erased.

The Act also stipulates that:

- Appropriate security measures shall be taken against unauthorized access to, or alteration, disclosure or destruction of, personal data and against accidental loss or destruction of personal data (Peckitt, 1989).

The Act emphasizes that the degree of security expected of a data user is related directly to the nature of the personal data and the degree of harm caused by loss, alteration, disclosure or destruction. Users are specifically liable for the physical security of the data, the security of the software system and the reliability of staff having access to the computer.

There are exemptions to the Act. In addition to exemption for the private domestic computer user, there are various governmental exclusions – the police, judiciary, revenue services, public data including the electoral roll, and certain financial services. The following classes of data are specifically excluded from the Act:

- payrolls
- pensions
- accounts
- statistical and anonymous research data
- social services data
- health data of certain sorts
- records held under professional legal privilege (Peckitt, 1989).

All health professionals have a responsibility to ensure that they are clear about whether or not any data they keep in personal or professional databases is kept legally and within the terms of the Act. Details of registration under the Act are available from the Data Protection Registrar, Springfield House, Water Lane, Wilmslow, Cheshire SK9 5AX.

Example software: **Paradox 3 SE (Borland)**

The Paradox in the name of this program is that the program combines power with simplicity of use. This certainly seems to be the case. It is easy to have a database up and running in 15 minutes. The program is easily installed onto your hard disk and then it is ready to use. It comes

> **Computing Tip 15**
>
> **Try before you buy**
>
> Although, on the surface of it, one computer is very much like another, in practice they vary quite a lot. Keyboards, in particular, are very personal things. You may like one sort and hate another. The quality of reproduction on the monitor can also vary from computer to computer. Try, if you can, to see and try out the computer you want, before you buy it. Try to avoid 'buying blind'.

complete, not with a huge handful of manuals, but with a very practical book called *The ABC's of Paradox*. Rather than having to delve into the depths of a complicated manual, the manufacturers supply a commercially available bestseller on the product. I found this to be both refreshing and attractive. Too often, programs are spoilt by their impenetrable manuals. To be able to sit down and read a book about the product is a real gain.

Paradox relies heavily on a tabular structure. Like all databases, you first have to get to grips with the notions of forms and fields. A form is a single page of data. A field is a single element of data within that single page. Imagine an address book. One complete name and address entry would be a form, whilst each line of the name and address (name, street, town, etc.) would be a field. With Paradox, you decide on your fields, fill them into columns across the screen, press F2 to complete the field-making element of the program, then enter your data.

The program accepts both words and numbers and is able to run a variety of mathematical functions on its fields. It also has extensive searching facilities. The relational element of the program means that you can look up data from more than one database. For example, you may be a college principal who keeps one database containing the names and addresses of your students. You may keep another database containing those students' examination marks. The relational feature allows you to draw on the 'marks' database from within the 'student' database. Relational databases are the most powerful of all databases and this feature is worth exploring in some detail once you have got the hang of designing forms and entering data.

The more expensive version of Paradox may allow you even more sophistication but the SE version is likely to satisfy most people's needs and wants.

Computing Tip 16

Keep it simple

Simplicity is genius, particularly when it comes to desktop publishing and wordprocessing. Just because your program has 30 different sorts of fonts, don't be tempted to use them all. When you plan hand-outs, posters or other graphical work, make sure that you use only two fonts. Also, avoid excessive use of pictures, columns and other 'details'. Simpler wordprocessing and desktop publishing usually looks far more professional than does the more complicated sort.

Example software: **DataPerfect (WordPerfect UK)**

DataPerfect is a relational database which is both powerful and likely to meet most people's needs. It will be ideal for people who are already using WordPerfect as many of the keystrokes are common to both programs.

DataPerfect is a fixed form database. That is to say that you first have to work out the structure of your data before you store it away. Units of data are stored in fields. Thus, typical fields in a bibliographical database would be these:

Field one: Author
Field two: Date of publication
Field three: Title
Field four: Publisher

Fields of this sort must usually be of a predetermined length. You must allocate a certain amount of space to each field before you start entering your information. The DataPerfect manual is excellent on this point. It suggests that you first sit down with a pad of paper and draw out your data entry format before you switch on your computer. This is an excellent idea. It is also a good idea to read the manual for this program. DataPerfect may be powerful but it is not particularly intuitive to use. Help is always at hand, though. Pressing F3 brings up context-sensitive help wherever you are in the program.

The program uses its own jargon to describe its features. Each 'page' of information is called a 'panel' and the data fields are contained within such a panel. You can link one sort of panel to another sort and thus open up other 'pages' of data. For example, in your bibliographical database, the first panel may contain the fields described above. You will have at your disposal all the information you need to enable you to find a full reference to go at the end of your essay. However, you could link this panel with another which contained a full description of the contents of the book. You could also link to another panel which contained quotes from any given book. In this way, the program really comes into its own. Through a series of linked panels, it is possible to access huge amounts of carefully structured information both quickly and easily. The worst part is planning out the database in the first place.

As with other WordPerfect programs, DataPerfect is very well packaged and contains an excellent and detailed alphabetical reference guide alongside the workbook mentioned above. It also comes with a cardboard template which sits just above the function keys to enable you to find the right keys to set up and access the program.

One other factor makes this program stand out from other database programs. Most others limit the amount of information that you can put in any given field. Often, this is as little as 250 characters. You have no such limitations with DataPerfect, which can contain up to 32 000. You are unlikely to run out of space with this program and could easily file away lengthy interview transcripts or reports. This may be a deciding factor when comparing various database programs. I know of no other commercial database that has an upper limit of this magnitude.

Example software: **Memory Mate (Broderbund)**

Memory Mate is a free form database program. Most other sorts of database programs are what are known as fixed form. With those, you first have to decide on the format of the information you are going to store. If, for example, you use a fixed form database to store all of your bibliographical references, you first have to decide on an order for each of the elements of your references. Thus you tell the program that in one column you will always list authors' names, in another you will always list dates of publication and in another, the titles. The free form database does away with the need for this or any sort of structure. All you do is call up the program, type in your notes, your bibliographical reference or whatever. You can type as much as six pages of notes and then save them as a single 'item'. To recall that item at a later date, all you have to remember is one or more words contained in it. Thus, you do a search on the word 'counselling' and up come all the notes and items in which you have used that word. Then, you can browse through your notes and items at your leisure. Once you have found the note you want, you can even paste it straight into your wordprocessor, and vice versa. If you are writing a paper for a course and hit a purple passage, you can pull out the best sentences, save them into Memory Mate and recall them at a later date. If you are writing an essay or a paper you can quickly marshal all your references at the end of your working session.

The lack of the need to structure your input into Memory Mate is one of its strongest features. There really are few boundaries. Names and addresses of friends can be entered straight after two or three paragraphs from your essay. Then you can put in some references and leave yourself a note about the letters you have to write. All of this material goes straight into the program. The entries can be as long or as short as you like. As long as you can recall a word or two from the entry, you are guaranteed to find it again – and quickly. Suddenly, the notepad and yellow stickers have become redundant. You have the equivalent of an almost endless reporter's notebook always to hand. You can even ask the program to remind you of things to be done on particular dates. In this way, it can be used as a diary and personal organizer.

Memory Mate is a 'terminate and stay resident' program. That is to say that you can load it into memory and it pops up over the other programs that you are using. You may, for example, be working in your wordprocessor and want to look up a reference. Pushing two buttons brings Memory Mate onto the screen, over your wordprocessor. You then find your reference and return to your wordprocessor.

The lack of structure also allows you great freedom in recalling the books and papers that you need. For example, you may remember that a particular book was published by Macmillan and was about client-centred counselling. The search facility will allow you to look it up using any one or more of those words. You no longer have to remember authors, dates, titles and so forth. As long as you have some recollection of what the book or paper was about, you are almost guaranteed to find it.

The program can be used in other ways. Recently, I used it to content analyse the data generated from some structured interviews that I had carried out. I transcribed the interviews straight into Memory Mate, making sure that each question and its answer formed a single note. It was then easy to recall all the answers to a particular question at the touch of a button. It was also possible to recall all the notes that contained particular words and phrases. The program allows you to work as you think. Just as you might experiment with organizing data that is written on paper by spreading your papers out all over the floor, so you can experiment with categories and notes in Memory Mate. It is versatile, adaptable and, best of all, easy to use.

Memory Mate is supplied on a single disk and is readily installed on any IBM compatible computer. It is easy to have it load straight into the memory of your computer when you switch on. In this way, it is always in the background and ready to be called up at any time.

Example software: **Info Select (Micro Logic)**

This is another excellent free form database and information organizer. It works as a 'terminate and stay resident' program and can be popped up over other programs. Data is entered into rectangles on the screen which are reminiscent of Post-it Notes. The size of the rectangles can be easily changed and each one can contain a considerable amount of text. Each rectangle can be used to hold a different piece of information. To search for data, all you do is type in any word that might be in the database and you are immediately presented with any rectangles that contain that word. Thus it is possible to explore the database in a variety of ways. Like all good programs of this sort, it is easy to use and very versatile.

Info Select has lots of potential uses for health care professionals including:

- the storage of bibliographic references;
- the analysis of qualitative data;
- the storage of odd notes and queries;
- the filing of names and addresses.

It can also be used as a diary, a reminder and alarm system and a hundred and one other uses. It is the sort of program that encourages you to think laterally.

OTHER DATABASE PROGRAMS

There is a variety of database programs on the market. A shortlist would include the following:

- Cardbox Plus
- Dataease
- Dbase
- Foxpro
- Masterfile
- R:Base
- Superbase

HEALTH CARE DATABASES: DATA ON A COMPACT DISK

As we noted in Chapter 2, the compact disk offers a means of storing a considerable amount of information in a compact medium. Compact disks store about 650Mb of information but this is 'read only': you can read the data of the disks (with the appropriate CD-ROM player) and you can use that data in your wordprocessor but you cannot write new information to the disk. The medium is ideally suited to supplying health care professionals with bibliographic information. A variety of CD-ROM is available and listed below are some of the ones most useful to health professionals. All of these and a wide range of other

CDs and CD-ROM drives are available, in the UK, from Microinfo Ltd, CD-ROM Division, PO Box 3, Omega Park, Alton, Hampshire GU34 2PG. The names in brackets refer to the publishers of these compact disks.

- **Aidsline** (Software Toolworks). This consists of information from several larger databases. Over 3000 journals have been scanned for inclusion in Aidsline. Subject coverage includes all aspects of the AIDS situation.
- **Biological Abstracts.** This is a research tool for those in the biological and biomedical fields. Entries include bibliographic citations and abstracts of current research reported in the biological and biomedical literature. Approximately 250 000 records are indexed per year.
- **The British Medical Journal 1986–1990** (Macmillan). Selections from one of the most important medical journals.
- **The Lancet 1986–1990** (Macmillan). This includes the complete text of articles from the *Lancet* between these years.
- **Martindale: The Extra Pharmacopoeia**. This is the complete text on disk and it is updated quarterly.
- **Oxford Textbook of Medicine** (Oxford University Press). This is the electronic edition of a standard text.
- **Healthcare Product Comparison System** (Dialog). This provides objective comparisons of brand name products covering all types of equipment used in health care from X-ray units to laser equipment.
- **Cumulative Index to Nursing and Allied Health Literature** (Cambridge Scientific Abstracts). The CINAHL provides access to virtually all English language nursing journals, publications from the American Nurses' Association, the National League for Nursing and primary journals in more than a dozen allied health disciplines. It also includes selected articles from approximately 3200 biomedical journals indexed in Index Medicus, from approximately 20 journals in the fields of health sciences, librarianship, educational and behavioural sciences, management and popular literature. Contains information from 1983 to the present and updated monthly.
- **Compact Library: AIDS** (Macmillan). This is a collection of clinical information on all aspects of AIDS treatment, research and patient management. This comprehensive disk includes the AIDS Knowledge

Base (an electronic textbook), the word for word text of articles from core medical journals including *AIDS, Journal of Infectious Diseases*, the *New England Journal of Medicine, Annals of Internal Medicine* and many more. Also included are thousands of bibliographical references to the literature from Aidsline and Medline and two new databases from the National Library of Medicine, Aidsdrugs and Aidstrials. All databases can be browsed or searched by key words and phrases.

- **Compact Library: Viral Hepatitis** (Macmillan). A comprehensive collection of information on hepatitis research from around the world, containing the Hepatitis Knowledge Base, a database of references to the hepatitis literature developed by physician editors. It also includes over 33 000 bibliographic citations and abstracts from Medline and the complete text of articles from core journals including the *New England Journal of Medicine*, the *Lancet* and the *British Medical Journal*. It is updated annually.

- **Medline** (Cambridge Scientific Abstracts). This provides access to worldwide biomedical literature and will be well known to many health care professionals. Contains Index Medicus, Index to Dental Literature and International Nursing Index. The field is indexed using the National Library of Medicine's controlled vocabulary, MeSH (Medical Subject Headings). All options feature two levels of searching (menus and command) with full MeSH explosion. Reference Update, a new enhancement to CSA's Medline, provides full tables of contents of over 1000 current journals up to 14 weeks before this information is available online. It is included with every update disk at no additional charge. Reference Update is updated weekly with key facts about new reports – title, author and citation data, including page numbers. When incorporated into Medline, Reference Update citations will be marked and remain on the disks until abstracted and published in Medline itself. Duplicate listings are then eliminated. I have used Medline on a very regular basis and find it to be a vital tool in literature searching in the health care field.

- **Micromedex – Computerized Clinical Information System** (Micromedex Inc.). Micromedex is an established publisher of evaluated patient care information. In 1974, Micromedex began publishing databases in conjunction with the Rocky Mountain Poison and Drug Center, Denver General Hospital and the University of Colorado

Health Sciences Center. The Computerized Clinical Information System (CCIS) is a database designed especially for health care professionals. CCIS includes up-to-date information on toxicology, drug therapy and acute care medicine. The TOMES Plus database provides medical and hazard data on thousands of chemicals. The database assists professionals concerned with the health and safety of people and the environment. Every 90 days subscribers receive updated data in compact disk format.

- **Oxford Textbook of Medicine** (Oxford University Press). This is the electronic edition of the standard text.

- **Sedbase** (Silver Platter). This contains the full text database of critical reviews of worldwide literature on clinically relevant side effects and interactions of all drugs currently in use. Topics covered include adverse drug reactions, drug interactions, drug toxicity, pharmacological or patient dependent factors associated with side effects and special risk situations. In all, it includes over 40 000 drug side effects and 4000 drug interactions. Sedbase is derived from the series *Meyler's Side Effects of Drugs* and *Side Effects of Drugs Annual*. It is updated semi-annually.

- **Year Book 1990 Edition** (CMC Research Inc.). This CD contains the combined 1988, 1989 and 1990 Year Books. Titles include: Dermatology, Diagnostic Radiology, Drug Therapy, Emergency Medicine, Family Practice, Medicine, Neurology and Neurosurgery, Obstetrics and Gynaecology, Paediatrics, Psychology and Applied Mental Health, Oncology, Cardiology, Critical Care, Infectious Diseases, Infertility, Orthopaedics, Sports Medicine and Surgery.

- **PsycLit** (Silver Platter). This series of compact disks contains citations to over 1300 journals in psychology and the behavioural sciences. Compiled by the American Psychological Society, the database provides coverage from 1974 to the present. Topics covered include all aspects of psychology, as well as behavioural aspects of education, medicine, sociology, law and management.

- **Sociofile** (Silver Platter). This is an index to and abstracts of the literature of sociology from 1800 journals published worldwide. It includes abstracts of journal articles published in *Sociological Abstracts* since 1974 and the enhanced bibliographic citations for relevant dissertations that have been added to the database since

1986. Also included is the Social Planning Policy and Developments Abstracts (SOPODA) database with detailed journal article abstracts since 1980.

- **Life Sciences Collection** (Cambridge Scientific Abstracts). This contains 18 subject oriented subfiles in the life and bioscience field, covering some 5000 core journals, books, serial monographs, etc. Over 98 000 abstracts are added each year and the collection is updated quarterly.

These databases of information for health care professionals illustrate the way in which the computer can aid workers in all parts of the health care field – but particularly, perhaps, researchers, writers and academics. These compact disks will be particularly useful to libraries in health care colleges and colleges of medicine and this listing can also be used for decision making in purchasing departments of libraries. It can also aid health care professionals who want to recommend purchases within their libraries. It is not until we know what is available in the database world that we can make informed choices. The listing above is not exhaustive but it may give some indication of the breadth and depth of material that is available.

Reference update

This is not data on a compact disk but on standard floppies. Reference Update regularly scans over 1200 newly published major journals of biology and medicine, indexing references to important new articles and papers many weeks before similar references appear in online databases such as Medline. The system is based on the tables of contents of the journals and indicates in each case the availability of full abstracts of the papers cited. Users may request copies of the articles by fax or, alternatively, the system will automatically print a 'reprint request' postcard with the author's name and address. Special postcards are available for purchase at a nominal cost. Where circumstances permit, online access to the abstracts is also available. Citations can be transported to an associated bibliographic management software package – Reference Manager – which enables downloading of references. Users with alternative database management software can automatically create a Medline formatted ASCII file for importation to their own database. There is also a Reference Update DeLuxe Abstract Edition service available which includes a full abstract with each citation. Both of these bibliographic reference database services are also available from Microinfo Ltd.

FURTHER READING

Sigel, C. (1989) *The ABC's of Paradox*, Sybex, San Francisco, distributed by Computer Manuals Ltd, 50 James Road, Tyseley, Birmingham B11 2BA

This book, with the wonderfully odd title, is of obvious interest to anyone who uses the Paradox series of database programs. It is also an example of the excellent 'how to do it' books published by Sybex. Like all of their books, it is clearly laid out, with plenty of examples from practice. It is also well illustrated with 'screen dumps' or pictures of how things will look on the screen.

The book covers fundamentals, such as explaining what a database is. It then tells you how to install Paradox and how to get started. Paradox, although an extremely powerful program, is also an easy one to get up and running. Later chapters deal with entering data, searching and sorting the database. There is also plenty of information on how to produce reports and how to import and export data. Oddly enough, the book is also a useful introduction to the whole idea of databases, although only Paradox users are likely to want to buy it. If you see it in the library, however, and still haven't decided on what program to buy, this book will offer you some useful information to help you make up your mind.

7 Other software for health care professionals

So far, we have seen how wordprocessors and databases can be useful in working with words and records. In this chapter, the focus is on other sorts of software that can be of value to any health care professional.

SPREADSHEETS

A spreadsheet offers you a giant 'rows and columns' program. The screen of a spreadsheet program looks like this on start-up:

	A	B	C	D
1	This is a 'cell'			
2				
3				
4				

Figure 7.1 A typical spreadsheet layout.

Each row of the spreadsheet is numbered and each of the columns has a letter allocated to it. The rectangle that those letters and numbers define is called a cell. Each cell can contain numbers or words and, used with numbers, the spreadsheet offers a powerful numerical computing tool. Most spreadsheet programs allow you to work with a potentially massive number of rows and columns. Many of the larger ones (and the smaller ones, come to that) will allow you a maximum of 256 columns and 8192 rows. Clearly, the size of the monitor screen limits the number of rows and columns that can be seen at any one time but all spreadsheet programs allow you to jump to a particular area on a larger spreadsheet and some allow you to view two or more parts of the rows and columns matrix at any given time. Most programs also have graphing, bar chart and histogram facilities.

Anyone who is used to working with figures will know the value of being able to work with rows and columns. Most figure work can be usefully represented in this way. Spreadsheet programs can thus be used for at least the following functions:

- general accounting;
- simple and complex arithmetical and mathematical calculations;
- analysis of quantitative research data, including frequency counts;
- cost-benefit analysis.

What is less frequently documented is that the rows and columns formulation of spreadsheets can also be put to good use with words and figures and even with just plain words. Here are two examples. Figure 7.2 illustrates how a spreadsheet program can be used to record off-duty in a hospital, clinical or community setting. Figure 7.3 demonstrates the spreadsheet program's use as a method of recording bibliographic data. In fact spreadsheets are often useful as databases. Their cells can be sorted alphanumerically and searches for specific words or strings of words can easily be carried out. Figure 7.4 illustrates the use of a spreadsheet for collating the data collected by questionnaire. In the example used here, respondents were asked questions of the following Likert-type:

Spreadsheets

Question 4. All health care professionals should have computing skills

Strongly agree	Agree	Don't know	Disagree	Strongly disagree	Leave blank
1.	2.	3.	4.	5.	

Thus, each response to each question can be tagged as either a '1', a '2', a '3', a '4' or a '5'. This sort of data is ideally suited for collation within a spreadsheet. All the responses to all of the questions can be listed in the spreadsheet and then frequency counts can easily be calculated to illustrate how many respondents offered particular sorts of responses to particular questions. The results of such a frequency count can then be graphed or drawn as a bar chart.

Spreadsheets are one of the most versatile of computer programs and most health care professionals are likely to benefit from owning or using one. Their benefit goes far beyond their use as simple 'balance

	A	B	C	D
1	27th May 1993	Cedar ward	Oak ward	Elm ward
2	Morning Shift			
3	Senior nurses	1	0	1
4	Primary nurses	4	3	4
5	Associate nurses	2	4	4
6	Student nurses	4	0	2
7	Nursing assistants	2	4	2
8				
9	Afternoon Shift			
10	Senior nurses	1	1	1
11	Primary nurses	2	2	3
12	Associate nurses	2	3	1

TOTALS:

Figure 7.2 Example of the use of a spreadsheet program for off-duty.

	A	B	C	D
1	Bibliographical Database			
2	Author	Year	Title	
3	Aaronson, R.	1992	Clinical Psychology	
4	Andrews, P.	1986	Caring for the Whole Person	
5	Andrews, P.	1989	Spiritual Aspects of Care	
6	Blackmore, D.	1988	Community Psychiatry	
7	Brown, D.J.	1978	How to Prescribe	
8	Mathews, R.	1992	Surviving Stress	
9	Newbury, L.	1990	Treating Neuroses	
10	Palmer, D.B.	1993	The Idea of a New Hospital	

Figure 7.3 Use of a spreadsheet program for a bibliographical database.

	A	B	C	D
1		Question 1	Question 2	Question 3
2	Respondent 1	1	2	3
3	Respondent 2	3	3	3
4	Respondent 3	2	4	1
5	Respondent 4	5	4	1
6	Respondent 5	5	4	2
7	Respondent 6	4	4	3
8	Respondent 7	3	3	5
9	Respondent 8	1	2	5
10	Respondent 9	1	2	1

Figure 7.4 Use of a spreadsheet program for the collation of questionnaire data.

sheets'. They can also help with 'what if' projections. It is quite possible to change one value in one cell, and to note its effect on all of the other figures in the spreadsheet – and particularly its effect on the bottom line. It is important, though, that large scale business and financial decisions are not made quickly on the basis of a spreadsheet computation. It is vital that all aspects of the spreadsheet figure work are checked before such decisions are made.

Checklist of spreadsheet functions

Features to look for in an advanced package include:

- automatic back-up facilities;
- emboldening, italicization and underlining facilities;
- automatic recalculation;
- cell copying facilities;
- block copying facilities;
- integrated graphics, including graphs, bar charts, pie charts and histograms;
- a wide range of mathematical functions;
- context-sensitive help screens;
- ability to import and export data in various formats;
- linear regression functions;
- ability to 'lock' specific cells and groups of cells so that new data cannot be added to them;
- ability to merge two or more spreadsheets;
- ability to work with more than one spreadsheet at a time;
- DOS and/or Windows compatibility;
- search facilities;
- page numbering;
- versatile printing features;
- ability to produce headers and footers;
- search and replace features;
- sorting of text and numbers;
- mouse support.

The most famous spreadsheet program is Lotus 1-2-3 and this set the trend for a particular style of layout for many spreadsheets. Many, for example, follow Lotus' lead in asking you to hit the '/' key to bring up context-sensitive menu systems.

Example software: **PlanPerfect (WordPerfect UK)**

PlanPerfect is a powerful spreadsheet program which allows you to set up, quickly, a small or a large spreadsheet. The data in that spreadsheet can then be charted in many types of graphs, bar charts, pie charts and other graphical formats. Again, this feature makes PlanPerfect ideal for the researcher. Learning the program is a straightforward process once you have got the hang of the idea of rows and columns. PlanPerfect also comes with a very useful workbook which enables you to learn almost all of the functions of the program on a self-teaching basis. Pressing F3 anywhere in the program brings you context-appropriate help through a series of on-screen help menus.

PlanPerfect works particularly well with other WordPerfect products such as the world-leading wordprocessing program WordPerfect. Data from the spreadsheets produced with PlanPerfect can be quickly transferred into WordPerfect, as can graphs, bar charts and other figures. It also comes with a very wide range of printer drives and so it is extremely likely that it is compatible with the printer that you use. If not, WordPerfect is very good at supplying unusual or new printer drivers very quickly. Generally, WordPerfect support is excellent.

Computing Tip 17

Using a mouse

If you use a mouse, investigate the various ways that you can use the 'double-click' feature. This often lets you bypass various program menus and can speed up the way you work in Windows.

Example software: **Quattro Pro SE (Borland)**

Quattro Pro SE offers all the usual spreadsheet facilities. You can add up columns, move data around, print out charts, graph your figures and perform complicated arithmetical and statistical functions. Overall, you are offered a range of 14 charts and graph types to choose from and it is simple to produce good looking pie and bar charts. Anyone who has to handle numerical research data is likely to appreciate this element of the program. It is very easy to try out a number of different ways of presenting data before printing out or transferring your findings to your wordprocessor.

The program is run by a series of pull-down menus which are easy both to access and to work with. If you prefer, you can operate the program with a mouse. This certainly makes working around a large spreadsheet a lot easier.

Another feature is the ability to work with more than one spreadsheet at a time. Rather like the pages in an accounts book, the program allows you to flip through a series of charts and to make comparisons between them. You can also run 'what if' calculations to see what differences changing particular values would make to an overall calculation. This will be of particular interest to those who manage budgets.

The program comes with an extensive manual which is both easy to read and useful. Overall, this is an excellent package and one which represents outstanding value for money. Anyone who works with figures is likely to find Quattro Pro SE useful. It is an up-to-date program with all the features that you are ever likely to need to manipulate figures and to design graphs. It makes good use of colour, offers you plenty of samples and examples and is generally an easy program to work with.

Other spreadsheet programs

There is a variety of other spreadsheet programs on the market. A shortlist would include the following:

- Lotus 1-2-3
- Excel

> **Computing Tip 18**
>
> **Using the 'block' function**
>
> The 'block' function is one of the most useful in most wordprocessing programs. Blocked text can have a variety of changes made to it. Learn all about the block function at an early stage of familiarizing yourself with your wordprocessor.

- Quattro Pro
- Supercalc

GRAPHICS

Graphics programs are the ones that let you draw or manipulate text in such a way as to produce diagrams, charts, graphs and other sorts of illustrations. Graphics programs are particularly useful if you want to prepare hand-outs, slides, overhead projector transparencies and illustrations for a research report. Many health professionals who have to pass on information to others will appreciate being able to do that in imaginative ways. A good graphics program will allow you to design your own presentations and diagrams and to edit them in very precise ways. You may want a graphics program to produce the following:

- graphs, pie charts or histograms for a research report;
- illustrations, diagrams and figures for papers, articles and books;
- slide shows for use in lectures or at conferences;
- 'flyers' which advertise a course, a service or a publication;
- overhead transparencies for use in lectures or presentations.

Many graphics programs come complete with sets of 'clip art'. These are predrawn pictures of a wide range of things from people to computers and churches to traffic signs. The user simply selects a piece of this clip art and drops it into his page of graphics. One of the problems of this approach is that clip art is now so widely used that many people recognize the graphics package that you have been using by your clip art! This can sometimes be a distraction at conferences. As a rough rule of thumb, avoid clip art that illustrates crowds, nurses, business men and (oddly) butterflies: these have all been overdone as illustrations in graphical presentations.

Checklist of graphics functions

A good graphics package will include all or most of these features:

- ease of use;
- mouse compatibility (you especially need this if you want to draw some freehand illustrations);
- ease of transfer of data from the graphics package to your word-processing program;
- reproduction of graphs, pie charts, bar charts and histograms from imported datasets;
- some predrawn charts to get you started;
- built-in spellchecking;
- screen preview so that you can see what the end product will look like;
- compatibility with a wide range of printers;
- ability to move 'objects' (pictures, blocks of text, etc.) around the screen;
- bullet lists;
- ability to reproduce a wide range of font shapes and sizes.

Graphics packages are available for use with both DOS and Windows. The advantage of Windows programs is that they make full use of WYSIWYG. As you work on the screen, you are able to see at once what your finished chart or diagram will look like. Perhaps the most famous graphics package (and, in my opinion, justifiably so) is Harvard Graphics. It is extremely well thought out and straightforward to use and is available both as a DOS and a Windows program.

The usual rule applies when working with graphics packages: keep it simple. Stick to one or, at the most, two fonts and change the size of them as necessary to produce the effects that you want. Do not put too many words on any one page or in a single diagram and go very easy on the use of clip art. It is very easy to produce amateurish examples of graphics presentations: they are often to be seen on noticeboards in colleges and university departments and stand out as 'home made'. The best diagrams and presentations probably go unnoticed as graphical works: instead, you are drawn to the information within them. And this is how it should be; the aim of producing a graphical presentation is to inform, not to stun.

Example software: **Applause 11 (Borland)**

Applause is a very powerful graphics package that can handle almost any sort of graphical requirement. Supposing, for example, that you needed to present a series of figures from a research project in a graph. Applause will not only produce the graph for you but it will also allow you to look at the data in other chart formats. You may, for example, experiment with pie charts and histograms. Supposing that you are giving a paper at a conference. Applause can offer you a slide show format or it can help you to produce illustrated overhead projection acetates.

The program runs under DOS and is best operated with a mouse – although this is not essential. It is not an intuitive program. I didn't find it easy to throw out the manual and to beaver away at the screen and keyboard. However, after a few basic skills are mastered, learning gets much easier.

Applause runs in three modes: chart, draw and present. The chart mode enables you to produce diagrams, graphs, tables and word illustrations. The draw mode offers a full range of both computer-generated and free-hand graphics. The present mode helps you to prepare your work for the printer, camera or plotter. You can at all times view your work in full graphical mode. That means that you can easily see what your chart or illustration will look like when it's printed out.

The program also comes with about 7000 pieces of up-to-date clip art. Examples, in Applause, include a range of borders, a series of arrows of various sorts and a huge range of simple pictures. The clip art selection also includes a range of useful 'backgrounds', scenic pictures which sit behind your main diagram or text. They not only personalize your presentations but they also make it more attractive.

The program comes complete with a well-written manual called *Applause 11: Up and Running* and a useful Quick Reference card. The manual offers a series of easy to follow lessons and a guided tour of the whole program. I did two of the lessons before finding that I could work the rest of the program out for myself. Screen-related help was always available from the F1 key.

A hard disk is essential for running Applause. It takes up about 5Mb once it is fully loaded. It does, however, offer a wide range of fonts including a selection of Bitstream fonts.

Computing Tip 19

Learn about DOS

Many programs on the market help you to bypass the DOS commands. Most wordprocessors and all menu programs are written so that you do not have to know very much about DOS at all. The basics of DOS are not particularly complicated. Take time to learn a few commands at a time. This will give you much more confidence in using your computer and will enable you to fix most of the common problems that can occur. Various books about DOS are recommended at the ends of chapters in this book.

Example software: **DrawPerfect (WordPerfect UK)**

This is a major graphic program from the makers of WordPerfect that enables you to produce a wide range of presentation aids, from overhead projector acetates and hand-outs to charts showing research findings and figures for articles and books. It also allows you to produce slides, graphs, charts, bar charts and freehand drawings.

DrawPerfect is likely to be very attractive to teachers, managers and anyone who has to produce professional reports and illustrations. It is easy to use, versatile and help is never far away.

On start-up, the user is presented with a working screen. Through manipulation of either mouse-driven icons or through the menu system, you are then free to develop charts, graphs, pictures, lists, presentation graphics and so on. These can all be easily customized and integrated with text. The program includes an impressive array of different sizes and shapes of typeface (or fonts). As always, the danger with this sort of program is that the new user can end up making a bit of a mess. Having all the facilities to produce graphical presentations does not mean that the user will automatically end up with a work of art. Simplicity is usually genius in these cases. It is probably best to work with one or two fonts and to produce very simple and uncluttered designs.

The program comes with a wide range of printer drivers. If there is not one for your particular printer (and this seems unlikely), WordPerfect is almost certain to be able to send you one.

DrawPerfect comes complete with a version of WordPerfect Shell. This is a menuing system which allows you to work with a friendly menu on starting up your computer. Instead of being faced with the implacable C prompt, you are given a choice of programs to run at the touch of a button. DrawPerfect is obviously one of those programs but you can tailor the menu system to include all of your other programs. You can also switch between the Shell, DrawPerfect and other WordPerfect programs. This means that you no longer have to close down one program to work with another; you can access another program from within DrawPerfect. This is particularly useful if you are designing a chart to illustrate an article or report. It enables you to cross-check details whilst developing your chart.

Printing out can take a long time. The output from the program, though, is excellent. If you are able to use a laser printer, it is difficult to distinguish the output from 'real printing'.

Other graphics programs

There is a variety of other graphics programs on the market. A shortlist of these would include:

- Aldus Freehand
- Aldus Persuasion
- Arts and Letters

- Corel Draw
- Freelance for Windows
- Micrographix Charisma
- PC Paintbrush

DESKTOP PUBLISHING

Many health professionals need or want to produce hand-outs, magazines, fly sheets and other sorts of output which would, in the past, have been printed. Whilst, as we have seen, simple graphical presentations can be produced with a graphics package, larger projects often need desktop publishing facilities. There is a range of documents that can be produced by such packages and these include:

- documents that are made up purely of text;
- documents composed of text and simple illustrations such as charts;
- complex documents containing multiple text styles and various types of illustrations;
- long documents containing lots of text and a considerable degree of structure (a 'how-to-do-it' manual would be an example here).

Checklist of desktop publishing functions

Whilst many top-end wordprocessing packages now contain desktop publishing features, a dedicated desktop publishing program can often do far more. Examples of the sorts of features that are often found in such programs include:

- the ability to change font size easily and consistently. If you are working on a magazine, for example, you may want to use a large font for article headings, a smaller font for subheadings and a standard sized font for the body of the text;
- the ability to work with a range of illustrations, diagrams and pictures;
- the ability to put text into columns;
- the ability to transfer text in and out of the program, to and from a wordprocessing program;

- the ability to devise 'style sheets', templates for keeping style consistent within a document. This is particularly useful if you are working on a very large document or you want to develop a 'house style' – a layout that is consistent over a period of time. If you look at any commercial magazine, you will find that the layout stays much the same over any given period of publication;
- the ability to work with a range of printers.

Budgett (1992) offers the following suggestions, amongst others, for the person who is considering buying a desktop publishing program (DTP):

- Determine whether you need a top-end DTP system with full professional design and output features, or a top-end wordprocessor with extensive text management and graphics compatibility. The difference in cost can be hundreds of pounds, so it doesn't make sense to pay for facilities you won't use.
- If you want to produce structured documents, check if text management and automatic tables of contents are supported. Even some of the top DTP packages lack the text capabilities of humble wordprocessors.
- Are you limited by your current hardware, or can you let your chosen software package dictate what hardware you need to buy? All DTP packages will quote a minimum hardware requirement and many will suggest a recommended set-up.
- Consider your preferred operating environment. Windows offers many advantages, including (in theory) easy printing, but ask yourself if it's worth upgrading your whole system for one application program.
- Will your chosen package give you adequate visual control? Not all WYSIWYG modes are readable, and the ability to zoom features may be limited.
- Check if a wide range of filters for wordprocessors is included. An ideal DTP package ought to work with your current wordprocessor – preferably in both directions – without regularly resorting to ASCII text.
- Check if your printer is adequately supported by integral or additional printer drivers accompanying the DTP software. 'Generic' drivers

will usually deliver the goods if you own a non-standard printer, but may come unstuck if you try to produce complicated documents (especially when artificially manipulating typefaces, tints and graphics).

Example software: **PagePlus for Windows (Serif (Europe) Ltd)**

This is a straightforward, economically priced and easy to use desktop publishing program that has a host of useful features. It is pasteboard based and allows full rotation of text and images, which makes it ideal for the production of hand-outs, flyers, small posters, headed notepaper and teaching aids. PagePlus produces output on almost all printers including dot matrix, ink-jet and laser. It has fairly comprehensive import and export features so that you can import your text from your own wordprocessor or send files to it. Over 100 clip art images are supplied with the program and so is a Pantone colour licence which means that if you have colour printing facilities you will get an accurate representation of colours on the screen.

Type size can be adjusted 'on the fly' between 4 and 250 points which means that type size can range from the tiny to the huge. Seventy scalable fonts are supplied with the program. Scalable fonts, as the name suggests, means that you can tailor your type size to suit the project you are working on. The program also allows you to expand, condense, slant and rotate words both on the screen and in the final, finished project. As with most Windows-based programs, this one is easy and intuitive to use and should be ideal for the health professional who wants to produce professional looking hand-outs, booklets and similar projects.

Example software: **TypePlus (Serif (Europe) Ltd)**

This is an excellent Windows program that does a small number of things very well indeed. It allows you to type a heading or a few lines of text and then play with those words simply by clicking buttons. You can, for example, change font sizes, switch the text to bold or italics, switch between black on white text or white on black. Nothing very special, so far. But, much more than this, you can change the look of the text dramatically. You can curl it, have the beginning of the line in large text, tapering to small at the end of the line. You can make the text sit as a half or full circle and so on. All this makes it an ideal program for preparing small elements of desktop published documents. You may use it, for example, for preparing a letterheading or an unusual banner in a fly sheet. Once you are happy with your creation, you click a button and save the whole thing to a Windows clipboard. You are then able to paste the element straight in to any other Windows program – a desktop publishing or wordprocessing package, for example.

This is the sort of program that is so simple to use and so entertaining that you can easily waste hours just experimenting with it. It is very reasonably priced and highly recommended.

Other desktop publishing programs

There is a variety of desktop publishing programs on the market. A shortlist would include the following:

- Adobe Illustrator
- Avagio
- Deskpress
- Express Publisher for Windows
- Express Publisher
- Freedom of the Press
- MS Publisher for Windows
- Pagemaker
- Ventura

BUYING SOFTWARE

You can buy software from a variety of sources. First, it is available in High Street shops. When it is bought this way, the customer usually pays full price for it. It is also possible to buy programs through the post from a variety of direct-selling dealers. This is often a much cheaper way to buy and most direct dealers' prices are way below the 'authorized' price. Finally, it is also possible to buy American versions of well established software directly from the USA. This is usually identical to the British version except when programs contain spell-checkers and thesauruses. Then, the American versions obviously contain American spellings. However, these can usually be edited out by the purchaser, but check this facility before you buy directly from the USA. Delivery from American companies is surprisingly quick. I have ordered software from the USA over the phone using a credit card and received the program within four days. However, you really need to know exactly what you want and need before you order in this way. Also, software companies may not allow you to register American software in the UK.

On the issue of registration, always register yourself as a user once you have bought a new program. All this normally entails is your filling in a card and sending it back to the company that produced the software. As a registered user, you are usually entitled to considerable phone-line support and often allowed to purchase upgrades of programs as and when they become available, at reduced prices.

No program stays current for very long. Some companies bring out new versions of programs about twice a year, some less frequently. You clearly have a choice: stay with the version of the program that you know or move up to the new version. If you do upgrade, you have to buy the new version – few companies supply upgrades free of charge. Jones (1992) suggests the following pros and cons of upgrading programs, amongst others:

Pros

- Minor bugs in earlier versions are fixed.
- The new program will have new features.
- It will usually offer a better presentation.
- It will be faster.
- There will be an improved user interface.
- It will usually be more logical and consistent.

Cons

- A new selection of bugs may appear.
- How many new features are you likely to use?

- You will have to pay for the upgrade.
- The new version may not work with older hardware.
- It may need more memory.
- You may need to upgrade your operating system.
- Data files in your present version may not be compatible with the new.

Apart from these pros and cons, it should also be noted that you are likely to have invested considerable time in learning you program. Any upgrade may mean relearning. Whilst most upgrades do not radically change the whole program, sometimes they do. This is particularly true of DOS versions of programs that are upgraded to Windows version. You may find yourself faced with what looks like a totally new program. On the other hand, most people like to keep up to date. The more you read about a new version of a program that you use, the more likely you are to want to upgrade to it! For better or worse, I have found that I have always upgraded my wordprocessing program as new versions have become available. Each time I have upgraded, I have said to myself that I would settle down with this version. This has been true . . . until the next version has come along!

FURTHER READING

Peckitt, R. (1989) *Computers in General Practice*, Sigma Press, distributed by Computer Manuals, 50 James Road, Tyseley, Birmingham B11 2BA

This is a useful book for anyone in the health professions who is beginning to work with computers. Although aimed specifically at GPs, it will also be of value to health care professionals who need to set up record systems, databases or any sort of larger scale installation. The book covers choosing a system and setting it up. It even starts from unpacking the box the computer comes in. This may sound like overkill but anyone who is new to computers and who has been faced with two or three large cardboard boxes filled with computer parts will appreciate it. This approach to beginners is refreshing. Too many computing books assume that the person reading them will already be able to start up the machine and call up programs. Even the manuals that are supplied with computers often assume this. There are very few books aimed at the absolute beginner.

The volume also has chapters on developing medical databases, data security and protection and has a detailed section on the Data Protection Act which will be of interest to anyone who needs to keep notes about other people. Also covered are training methods, using a wordprocessor, spreadsheet and graphics packages. All of these issues are related directly to the health care field.

The author does not claim to be a computer expert but a person who uses computers regularly in his own practice. Like some of Wagner's operas, the book would have been improved by a good sub-editor as it is not always clearly laid out. Towards the end of the book, the author jumps from one topic to another in an annoying way. Having said all that, there is a lot that is useful here. One of the strengths of the book is that it is directly related to health care. Whilst there are many books aimed at the computer user, few have this specific focus. There are lots of ideas that other health professionals will be able to use.

8 Shareware

Shareware is quite different to commercial software. It has a unique marketing strategy. A shareware program is distributed free of charge (although a charge is usually made for the disks and the handling). The idea is that you first try the program and then, if you like it, you send away a registration fee to use the program. In the first instance, you usually have between 30 and 90 days to try out the program before you register it. Further, during this time, you are encouraged to make copies of the program for your colleagues and friends. Then, the same principles apply: they are allowed to try out the program and then send off to become registered users if they find it useful.

ADVANTAGES

The advantages of the shareware approach are many for the home personal computer user. First, he or she gets a chance to try the program before making a financial commitment to it. Second, the registration fees for shareware are considerably cheaper than the cost of most commercial programs. Also, the quality of shareware programs is improving all the time and some of the best are easily the equal of commercial software. Finally, shareware offers you the easy approach to learning more about computer programs and enables you to explore a variety of methods of working with data that would not have been possible if you had to rely on buying commercial packages.

The names and addresses of shareware distributors are available in any of the monthly computer magazines. Such magazines often include one or two shareware programs on a 'free' disk attached to the front cover. Anyone who is contemplating buying software – or hardware, come to that – should read one or two of the monthly computer magazines. There are lots to choose from and all of the bigger newsagent chains carry them.

HISTORY OF SHAREWARE

Shareware, freeware, and user-supported software are all terms used to describe a relatively new phenomenon in the PC world. It began in March 1982 when the late Andrew Fluegelman introduced PC-TALK (a communication program). For several years before this, computer user groups and bulletin board systems had created a network of communicating personal computers allowing users of compatible systems to take advantage of each other's knowledge. These systems were in place when Fluegelman realized that there was no software available that would allow incompatible systems to communicate. After trying to modify available programs he decided to write his own.

The program allowed any computer to communicate with any other computer via the telephone. It worked so well that some friends suggested he do something public with it. Rather than follow the traditional publishing route, Fluegelman decided to send his program out for free, encouraging people to copy and distribute it and asking people to make donations if they liked it. In return, he would supply them with upgrades. Within a week of making the program available he received his first order. Very quickly he had to replace his post box with a larger one and buy a few more disk drives. Shareware was born.

Around the time of Fluegelman's success, a former IBM employee, Jim Button, had successfully converted an AppleSoft BASIC program called EASY-FILE, that he had written as a hobby, to the then new IBM PC. Out of a simple desire to share a good thing, he distributed the program among friends and colleagues. Friends shared with friends, associates with associates and soon hundreds were using the program.

Problems soon developed trying to notify users when fixes or improvements became available, such as how to identify serious users who needed or desired the upgrades. Mr Button decided to place a message in the program encouraging people to use and distribute the program and to send a donation of $10 if they wanted to be included on his mailing list. The first person to respond telephoned almost immediately mentioning another program, PC-TALK, that had a similar message.

The two original Shareware authors got together and decided to refer to each other in their disk documents. EASY-FILE became PC-FILE and the requested donation became $25. In May 1983 *PC World* magazine gave PC-FILE a rave review.

Three months later, Bob Wallace introduced PC-WRITE and with it, the idea of commission shareware. To encourage people to distribute and register his program, Mr Wallace's company (Quicksoft Inc.) sends each registered user a copy of the program with its own unique registration number. The newly registered user can then distribute his or her personalized copy and each time someone else registers a copy Quicksoft will pay the owner a commission. PC-WRITE is without question a super program, but there can be no doubt that commission shareware has played a significant part in its success.

Since its introduction by these pioneers, shareware has evolved into a competitive marketing alternative. Million dollar companies (like Buttonware and Quicksoft Inc.) and literally hundreds of entrepreneurial authors have been offering commercial quality software and support at an unbeatable price.

The Association of Shareware Professionals

In April 1987 the Association of Shareware Professionals (ASP) was established. ASP members are programmers and vendors who subscribe to a uniform code of ethics and are committed to the shareware method of marketing. The ASP's standards for its members are:

Programming Standards

The program must meet the ASP's definition of 'shareware'. It may not be a demo program with a major feature disabled, nor a time limited or otherwise 'crippled' program.

Documentation Standards

Sufficient documentation must be provided to allow the average user to try all the major functions. Discussion of the shareware concept and of registration requirements is done in a professional and positive manner.

Support Standards

Members will respond to people who send registration payments as promised in the program's documentation. At a minimum, the member will acknowledge receipt of all payments. Members will establish a procedure for users to report, and have acknowledged, matters such as bug reports, and will describe such means in the documentation accompanying all versions of the program. The author will respond to written bug reports from registered users when the user provides a self-addressed, stamped envelope.

Known incompatibilities with other software or hardware and major or unusual program limitations must be noted in the documentation that comes with the shareware (evaluation) program.

Shareware is not just a novel idea. It is a real solution to the program author's distribution problems and the software consumer's high prices. It's simply great for everyone, but will work only if authors keep their promises and consumers pay for the products they use. So if you like the shareware concept, support it and register programs you use.

EXAMPLES OF SHAREWARE PROGRAMS

A wide variety of types of shareware programs is available. These include programs in the following groups:

- artificial intelligence programs;
- business software;
- database programs;
- data sets of various sorts;
- desktop management programs;
- educational programs;
- engineering and electronics software;
- games;
- graphics programs;
- statistics and maths programs;
- utility programs for managing your computer and your hard disk;
- programs specifically written for Windows.

Examples of specific shareware programs are described briefly in Appendix 3 of this book.

> **Computing Tip 20**
>
> **Trim your programs**
>
> If you are short of hard disk space and if you know your programs well, comb through the files in that program's subdirectory and delete unnecessary files. Many program manuals will list the files that are contained in a program and will tell you which ones are essential and which ones are optional. Many programs, for example, automatically load a range of 'printer drivers', many of which you will not need to use. Only erase files that you know are unnecessary. It is a good idea to create a subdirectory called TEMP on your hard disc. Before you erase any files from any programs, move them into this subdirectory. If, at the end of the week, your program has not 'missed' the files, you can erase them. You may also want to put certain rarely used data files in this subdirectory (after you have backed them up to floppies). If you have not used the files after a month, consider erasing them from the hard disk. The TEMP directory is a 'holding' directory for files that are about to be removed but it serves as an additional fail-safe device.

FURTHER READING

Gardner, D.C. and Beatty, G.J. (1992) *Windows 3.1: The Visual Learning Guide*, Prima Publishing, Rocklin, California, distributed by Computer Manuals, 50 James Road, Tyseley, Birmingham B11 2BA

There is an increasing amount of shareware now available for the Windows environment. This is the ideal handbook to enable you to learn Windows in easy stages. One of the most impressive features of this book is the quality of its illustrations. Each page contains a number of high quality screen shots which graphically illustrate the points under discussion. All aspects of setting up and running Windows are covered in this easy to use guide. Highly recommended for any health professional who is not yet using Windows or who wants to brush up.

9 Writing skills

At some point in their careers, all health care professionals have to write. Some enjoy it and others do not. Almost all health professionals are required to take educational courses throughout their careers. The 'front-end' model of education and training in the health care field is rapidly disappearing. The idea that you could undertake a training course – however lengthy – and then be set up for life is now recognized as an impossible one. We all have to keep up to date for the shelf life of knowledge is so short. Fortunately, computers offer an important tool for both improving writing and making the process of doing it easier.

WRITING WITH A COMPUTER

Writing straight to a screen takes a bit of getting used to. I have met people who write things out in longhand and then type it all into the wordprocessor. This is understandable but it misses the point of computing. Writing straight to the screen saves time. The time that is saved can be used to improve what you have written. The wordprocessor is almost infinitely flexible: it can let you polish and improve your work almost endlessly. This, of course, can be a drawback as well as a strength. You have to stop somewhere. Too much polishing can produce staid and tired prose. You have, then, to learn a certain balance. The best way is often to write drafts very quickly, then to edit more slowly and then to stop.

GENERAL PRINCIPLES OF GOOD WRITING

Writing skills vary considerably. The type of writing that you have to do will often determine the style. The style you use to produce a report

> **Computing Tip 21**
>
> **Working with more than one file at a time**
>
> Many wordprocessors allow you to open more than one data file at a time. Thus, you may be able to switch between a report you are writing and the chapter of a book you are also writing. To avoid confusion about which file you are in, set the defaults of your wordprocessor to show a different colour scheme for each of the different file screens. For example, in WordPerfect, I have the main screen showing yellow characters on a blue background and the 'second' screen showing yellow characters on a maroon background. This means that I always know which screen I am working on. Be particularly careful when showing the same file in both screens. It is easy to make changes to one version of your work and not to the other. It is also easy to erase the 'wrong' version. Some wordprocessors allow you to compare two versions of the same file and show you, graphically, the changes that have been made to either or both.
>
> All this applies particularly if you use a Windows-based wordprocessor. Windows allows you to open a large number of files at once and to switch between them very quickly.

about the clinical area in which you work will be quite different to the style you use for an academic thesis. There are, though, some basic rules of writing that apply in almost all situations. Robert Gunning (1968) offers ten principles of clear writing:

- Keep sentences short.
- Prefer the simple to the complex.
- Prefer the familiar word.
- Avoid unnecessary words.
- Put action in your verbs.
- Write like you talk.
- Use terms your reader can picture.
- Tie in with your reader's experience.
- Make full use of variety.

- Write to express, not impress.

It is worth considering each of these in turn and the reader is also referred to Gunning's book. It is a readable and important analysis of how to write well.

Keep sentences short

Writing short sentences and short paragraphs is the key to good writing. Many people writing essays and manuscripts for the first time tend to write sentences that are far too long. Many are joined by 'and' and by colons and semi-colons. The computer is an ideal instrument for making sure that you keep sentences short. First, write your piece, then go back and edit. As you edit for the first time, pay attention only to the length of the sentences and prune as you go. You will be surprised at how many sentences you can shorten.

On the other hand, do not write too many short sentences. Lots of them can make for a 'staccato' style of writing (and reading). Aim at most of your sentences being short ones but at some of them being longer. A good 'style checking' program can help you with this aspect of writing and Grammatik, reviewed on pp. 159–60, will help to detect your longer sentences.

Prefer the simple to the complex

It is important not to try to impress. You reader will not appreciate it. Stick to ordinary words and do not try to confuse. As one lecturer at university told me, 'Anyone who has anything interesting to say will not risk being misunderstood'. Some students on courses are tempted to use rather flowery language in the belief that it will sound 'academic'. Some academics are tempted this way too. This is fine if you are writing an academic monograph to be read by a handful of other people but most of us are not.

Prefer the familiar word

It is tempting to try to introduce unusual words into your writing. Some people use such words because they feel that they add interest to their writing. Others, as we shall see, do so to impress readers. Try to do neither of these things. All writing is a form of communication. As such, it is essential that the reader understands what he or she is reading. Familiar words are nearly always to be preferred to the more complicated or unusual.

Avoid unnecessary words

Try to cut out the 'howevers' and the 'neverthelesses'. Avoid qualifying adjectives with 'very' (as in, 'it is very important that student social workers . . .'). Especially avoid double qualification ('very, very'). Some writers almost unconsciously use a particular word too frequently (I, for some reason, have a soft spot for the word 'vital'). If you discover such words in your own writing, use the search and replace function of your wordprocessor and replace that word, throughout your paper or manuscript, with another. Better still, ring the changes and use a variety of words as replacements.

Put action in your verbs

Words like 'stop' and 'move' keep people reading. Try to make your writing active rather than passive. There is still a tendency in the academic world for everything to be written in the past tense. Try breaking that rule. Also, avoid clumsy sentence constructions such as 'The writer feels that . . .' or 'The current author acknowledges that . . .'. It is better to write 'I think that . . .'. After all, it must be clear that **you** are the writer or author.

Write like you talk

This statement itself is an example of 'writing like you talk'. More grammatically, it should be 'write as you talk'. Many people, when faced with writing, seem to lose the ability to express themselves as easily as they do in speech. Who would **say**, for example: 'I feel that it is of considerable importance that students in the health professions are offered the provision of open learning'? Probably no one. If you tend to write in this way, try clipping those sorts of sentences down like this: 'Students should be offered open learning facilities if they need them'. The test of whether or not you are observing this rule is to read out what you have written. If you wouldn't say it, don't write it.

Use terms your reader can picture

Try to use metaphors and illustrations that create pictures for the reader. Just because you are writing a report does not mean that you cannot 'illustrate' your writing in this way. Be careful, though. Make sure that you do not mix metaphors. This, apart from being grammatically wrong (which is not a big problem), causes all sorts of problems with imagery.

Don't highlight your own wit and humour. Wherever possible, avoid the 'screamer'. The screamer is the writing trade's name for the exclamation mark. If something is funny or ironic, the readers will notice. You don't have to rub their noses in it. If you do use an exclamation mark, only ever use one, never two or three.

Tie in with your reader's experience

People enjoy reading things that relate to their own experience. Illustrate what you write with small case studies or illustrations from life. Invite readers to think of their own examples of what you are talking about. At the same time, avoid rhetorical questions. It is irritating to read questions that seem to hang in the air without answers.

Make full use of variety

If you are writing an article for a journal, use checklists and boxed 'word illustrations'. This helps to break up large chunks of text. Look through any magazine that you have to hand. What you will find is that only the academic journals use continuous blocks of text. All the others use variety to keep the reader interested. On the other hand, don't use these devices for their own sake. Make sure that they add to the reader's understanding of your writing.

Write to express, not impress

Your aim should not be to show how clever you are. It should be to communicate your ideas to other people. This point seems to summarize all of the other ones. Many students, when they start to write essays for diploma and degree courses, think that they have to try to imitate the worst sorts of academic writing. Perhaps they read papers in fairly dull journals. Perhaps some of their lecturers talk in that way. Whatever the reason, the point is to stop writing in that fashion. Write simply, clearly and use the obvious word rather than the more complicated.

Avoid 'sic'

The word 'sic' is sometimes put in brackets after a direct quote from someone else's work. It is there to indicate that the current writer acknowledges that the passage is not quite right, grammatically or in terms of spelling or structure. The use of 'sic' can sound smug. It is best avoided if at all possible. There are times when you need to indicate that an unusual form of words was used. If you are writing up a research

---

Computing Tip 22

Preparing camera ready copy

Some publishers ask people who are writing for them to prepare camera ready copy. That means that the manuscript the author sends in is photographed and used as text in the final publication. Therefore the copy must be completely accurate and follow the publisher's style exactly. Make full use of 'style sheets' and similar functions in your wordprocessor to make sure that all of the layout of your text is consistent. Pay particular attention to the following:

- sizes of margins – in camera ready copy, these must be exact;
- spelling;
- style and size of subheadings;
- style of paragraphing;
- quality of final printout. Usually, only laser printing is acceptable for camera ready copy;
- quality of illustrations and diagrams.

Preparing camera ready copy is a painstaking job. You must make sure that the final printout is kept extremely clean as even a hair can show up in the final pages of the published book! Make sure that you have detailed instructions from the publisher and be prepared to have to make a considerable number of corrections to a manuscript that you think is perfect.

report that calls for direct quotes from interviews, then you need to use the respondent's own words.

PARAGRAPH LAYOUT

Make an early decision about how you will show paragraphs in any documents that you write. There are at least two options here:

- Indicate the start of a new paragraph by indenting every paragraph except the first under a heading (for an example of this, see the layout of this book). If you use this format, you do not put two 'hard returns' between paragraphs.

- Indicate the start of new paragraphs by leaving two 'hard returns' between them.

The examples below indicate the two options. Do not simply press the return key at the end of your last sentence and then start a new paragraph. This will make your text appear to have no paragraphs in it at all. Choose one or other of the above options and stick to it. The only time that you may have to change your style is if you are asked to prepare camera ready copy for a publisher to an exact specification (see Computing Tip 22).

Examples

Paragraph styling one

Here, you simply press the RETURN button twice between paragraphs. This used to be the standard way of preparing paragraphs in early computer work. Increasingly, the style below has replaced this 'block' style.

Here is the second paragraph, using this style. All that separates the two paragraphs is one empty line. The style offers a very 'clean' approach to preparing a manuscript.

Paragraph styling two

This is an example of paragraph layout using indentation. You indent the beginnings of each paragraph except the first under a heading or at the beginning of the piece.

When you use this style, use the TAB button to indent the paragraphs and never simply press the space bar five times. If you want to change the amount of indentation later, you can do so if you have used the TAB button. You simply change the default settings for the TAB button.

If you have inserted spaces with the space bar, you will have to change all of your indenting manually.

STYLE

This is the most difficult thing of all to define. Style is not content. It refers to the way in which words are put together. Like other sorts of reading, it is worth learning to read for style. This is easier with fiction than with non-fiction. Style is, however, present in non-fiction even if it is almost buried by the content. Too often, the style in non-fiction slips by us because we are caught up with the content. On the other hand, we do notice the style in that we readily categorize that book as 'bad' and this one as 'easy to read'. The hardest thing of all is to begin to notice your own style. There is something paradoxical here. If you work at developing a style, you are likely to lose it. You begin to turn out pieces that are self-conscious. Try, instead, to forget your own style but work away at getting the following things in order:

- sentence construction;
- paragraph construction;
- use of new metaphors;
- clear use of description;
- interesting reporting of research;
- ability to inspire the reader;
- enough 'padding' between facts to keep the reader reading.

The last point refers to the idea that we cannot keep offering the reader fact after fact. In between chunks of facts, we need to have a little relief. This can come in the form of criticism or commentary on what has gone before. Notice how other writers use this. Do not be tempted to pare down your style of writing so much that you leave out any sort of padding. On the other hand, be wary of page filling for the sake of it. Lecturers and tutors who have to mark essays will be very aware of students' attempts at such page filling. Take, for example, the following:

> Most of us, if we think about it, are caring by nature. It is essential that anyone in a caring or helping role feels warmth towards others. Warmth is an essential ingredient in the therapeutic relationship. Without it, the relationship can be sterile. Warmth brings a compassionate dimension to the caring role. Anyone who comes into the profession is likely to feel this way to start with. Professional training merely helps to build on this...

Managers are also famous for their use of page filling – and jargon. It is quite common to come across reports of this sort:

> Since the unit opened, the throughputs have exceeded those that had been expected. The way forward should be towards our making full use of staff potential in what can only be described as difficult times. We have faced continual cuts in manpower and in real-time equivalents. This has encouraged us to take a leaner long-term view. That fact must not blind us to the need to conceptualize client care in imaginative ways...

Baker (1987), in a book about sub-editing, discusses the following basic rules of style:

- Rewrite long sentences.
- Replace pompous or polysyllabic words with simpler ones.
- Make sure that the author's sentence construction is clear.
- Omit unnecessary adjectives and omit qualifications such as 'very'.
- Ensure that words are used precisely.
- Make sure that verbs are active.
- Make sure that the author uses metaphors correctly and sparingly.
- Replace jargon with a phrase in everyday use.

APPLYING THE PRINCIPLES TO WORDPROCESSING

Working with a wordprocessor, as we have acknowledged already, can be different from working with a pen and pad. There is a number of tips that can make writing easier with a wordprocessor. Some of these are itemized below. Try to standardize the way that you work so that your output is consistent. If you decide, for example, to use 2" margins when you write essays, always use 2" margins. Consider resetting the margin defaults to 2", so that every piece of writing you produce has 2" margins. This sort of standardization is important.

- As a rule, write quickly and edit later. One of the best things about wordprocessing (and possibly, also, one of its drawbacks), is that you can write your initial draft in any format and then go back and 'polish'. When you have to write on paper, the fact that you really will have to rewrite means that you are likely to take more time over what you write. The wordprocessor gives you much more freedom to experiment and to edit. There comes a time, of course, when you have to say 'enough!'. It is tempting to continue editing until you feel you have the perfect document. Such an aim is impossible. Settle for slightly less than best possible. At some point, just stop editing. Otherwise, the wordprocessor will work against you and you will take more time over your work than you did when you used a pen and pad. On the other hand, it is useful, occasionally, to return to working with a pen and pad. The change of medium can help you to pay much more attention to the craft of writing well.
- Many people write drafts on paper and then type out their work. Always write direct to the screen. To write in longhand first is to miss the point of wordprocessing which is that it allows you complete freedom to write and edit . . . and then to edit some more.
- Work in single spacing when you work at the keyboard. Although your final output will usually be in double spaced lines, use single spaced lines to work with on your screen. Double line spacing on the monitor means that you effectively halve the amount of text you can see on the screen at any one time.
- Try changing the speed of the cursor. If necessary, reset the speed according to the work that you are doing. If, for example, you are scrolling through long documents, set the cursor speed to high. If you are doing word by word or line by line editing, slow the cursor down. Not all wordprocessors allow you to change the speed of the cursor.
- Make full use of the block function of your wordprocessor. It is one of the most useful functions in the program. You can use it to erase,

edit, move, spellcheck, word count and so on. Experiment with the block feature until you are sure that you know all of the things you can do with it.

- Keep your work in small files. You do not need to keep the whole of a piece of work in one file. Large documents take time to work through. It may be better to split a large document into two separate files. If necessary, you can easily bring together the contents of two or three small files to make one larger one.

- Set the margin settings to 'wide' when working on large documents. This will mean that there are fewer words on each line on the screen. This will allow you to scan lines of text more easily. You can change the margin size back to normal when you have finished editing. Many wordprocessors cause words to be scrolled off the edge of the screen if your margin settings are too narrow. WordPerfect is an example of this sort of program.

- Make sure that you save your work to disk very frequently. Even if your program has an autosave function, the work that this saves will be deleted if you turn off your machine. Get into the habit of saving what you have written every time you stop to think for a few moments. Usually, the save function involves just one or two strokes of the keyboard. If it doesn't work as simply as this, make yourself a macro which assigns the save function to two keystrokes.

- Be consistent in your use of underlining, emboldening and italics. Don't mix the three. Settle for one type of emphasis and stick to it. If you use a laser printer, you can change the underlining key in your wordprocessor to show italics. In most cases, underlined text is 'translated' into italics when a piece of text appears in print. With laser printing, you can virtually do away with underlining altogether.

- Be consistent in your line spacing between ends of sections and new subheadings. As a rule, leave two lines between the end of a section and a new subheading. Then leave on line between the subheading and the text.

- Be careful about indenting paragraphs. Do not indent the first paragraph of a piece of work, nor subsequent first paragraphs under subheadings. After that, indent every paragraph. For an immediate example of both line spacing and indentation, look at the use of both in this book, which is laid out according to the standard rules governing page layout.

- Be consistent with your use of full stops and commas. It is not always necessary to use commas in a 'bullet' list (such as this one). If you do use them, use them consistently.
- Avoid mixing up different fonts on a page. It is not good practice to use all the different sizes of numbers and figures that your wordprocessor will allow. Keep to one or two sizes. As a general rule, 12 point is a good size font to use for everyday writing; and Times Roman is a clear and clean font if you have a laser printer. Fashions in typefaces come and go. At the moment, sans serif fonts (those without 'tails' on the letters) tend to be out of fashion (except, perhaps, for use in headings and subheadings). Times Roman seems to be something of a standard font. Here are examples of the three main types of font that you will come across in wordprocessing.

Courier. `This is the font that most nearly matches that of a typewriter. A number of dot matrix printers and a few laser printers can only print in this type of font. If you can, though, avoid it. If you had wanted to offer a typescript, presumably you would have used a typewriter.`

Times Roman. This is one of the most widely used fonts in the publishing world and is one of the easiest to read. Try to make sure that your wordprocessor and your printer can produce this sort of font.

Sans serif. Although this is clear and easy to read, it is probably best reserved for use in headings and for special effects. It is sometimes used as a 'modern' font in magazine production.

- Be careful over your use of graphics. If your wordprocessor can use clip art or predrawn pieces of illustration, use it very sparingly, if at all.
- If you can work in more than one document at a time and have a coloured screen, change the background colours in the second and third document screens. In this way, you are less likely to get muddled up about which document you are working on.
- If your wordprocessor has a thesaurus, use it regularly to give you ideas for different words. This can not only teach you words but it can freshen your writing.

- If you can, run off a draft 'hard' copy of your work before you submit it. It is often easier to spot typographical errors on the printed page than it is on the computer screen.
- Do not work for long periods at the computer. If you have to, work on different documents. It is a great strain to both eyes and posture if you work for hours on one document. Look away from the screen when the computer is busy working at a particular function. Get used to getting up and walking around the room at regular intervals. Take long coffee or tea breaks.
- When you start a session, take a look at what you worked on last. This allows you further scope for editing. It also puts you in the frame of mind for working. Starting from a completely blank screen can be a daunting experience.
- If you need to save small 'temporary' files of notes and fragments, give them unusual names. I call my temporary files 'PIG', 'CAT' or 'DOG'. In this way, I know, as I scroll through lists of files, that these are temporary. I know, too, that they are ones that I can delete as soon as I have used them. Their odd names make them stand out. The brevity of their names also means that it is difficult to mistype those names. If necessary, work out your own scheme for dealing with temporary files. You may prefer, for example, to use numbers and to call your files '1', '2', '3' and so on.
- Work on different parts of a long document at different times. If you are writing a long report or a book, do not feel that you have to work through it from cover to cover. It is often better to work in short bursts on different parts of a long document. On the other hand, this style of working can lead to a rather inconsistent style of presentation in the final document.
- Spellcheck and word count as you go. Keep a record of the number of words that you have written. This can help as a motivator when you feel you are running behind schedule. Keep a note of the date next to the number of words. Then you really can see the progress you are making (or not, as the case may be). I open up an entry in the pop-up, freeform database, Memory Mate, head it up and then keep a running account of the words I have written. An example of the entry for this book is illustrated in Figure 9.1. It allows me to call up 'Computing' at any time and to check how much I have written and how much I still have to write.

Computing book: word count
Chapman & Hall
Total word allocation: 70 000

Saturday 9 May 1992: 9719
Monday 10 May 1992: 12 251
Saturday 18 May 1992: 14 315
Sunday 19 May 1992: 16 673
Saturday 21 May 1992: 28 760
Sunday 22 May 1992: 29 858
Wednesday 27 May 1992: 35 048
Thursday 28 May 1992: 41 002
Friday 29 May 1992: 47 466
Saturday 30 May 1992: 49 550
Saturday 30 May 1992: 50 181

Figure 9.1 Example of a freeform database entry for keeping a word count tally.

TIPS FOR WORDPROCESSING WITH WINDOWS PROGRAMS

Windows-based wordprocessors allow you to see on the screen what will appear on the printed page. Because of their graphical user interface, they are usually slower than their DOS-based counterparts but can be more flexible. Here are some things you can do to speed up your Windows wordprocessing:

- Enter your text first and format the document later. This is a good, all-round tip. There is no need to work on the finer points of margin size and page layout until you have the bulk of your text on the screen. With Windows-based wordprocessors, the page layout is sometimes easier once you have typed your document. Also, you can experiment with the sorts of layout you may want to use.

- While you are typing, work with a larger than normal font. When you have finished your typing, revert to a more 'normal' font (10pt or 12pt are the most usual) for the final printout. If you do this, check through your document for layout before you print. A larger font, for typing, is easier on the eyes.

- If you type very quickly or like to work fast, consider working in draft mode. This is the non-graphical mode of the Windows wordprocessor and is not so attractive to look at and not WYSIWYG. It is, however, faster.

- Call up all the programs and **applets** (small Windows applications) before you start your wordprocessing session. Then, reduce the ones you are not currently using to icons. They will then be 'behind' your wordprocessing screen and available for use at the touch of the mouse. In some wordprocessing programs, you may want to start up the spellchecking, file finding and thesaurus features of the program in this way. This can make running these features a lot faster. On the other hand, do not have too many main programs working at any given time. If you fill up the memory of your computer with two or three large programs, you will find that your wordprocessor slows down to a crawl.

- Learn all about macros or short-cut features of your program. This can speed up your wordprocessing considerably. In WordPerfect for Windows, you can assign these macros to the button bar icon. One click on the button bar starts up the macro of your choice. Examples of macros that I have found useful for wordprocessing include ones that:

  — indent both sides of the margins. This is useful when you are using direct quotes in an essay or paper;
  — switch a document from single line spacing to double line spacing. Again, this is useful, at the end of an editing session, for preparing a paper for use as an essay or as a manuscript for publication;
  — start up a bullet list – such as this one. Such a macro is not all that easy to compose. I am always surprised that most wordprocessors don't have a bullet list feature as standard;
  — cut and/or paste blocks of text;
  — switch to another document screen or window;
  — call up a document, in another window, containing bibliographical

references. Such references can then be cut and pasted straight into the document in which I am working;
— spellcheck;
— word count;
— quit the program, saving the current document. This is a useful 'emergency' macro, for use when partners or children get sick to death of your working on the computer!
— call up a standard letter layout;
— strip extra spaces out of a document. This is a useful macro if you frequently import documents in other wordprocessing formats or in the universal standard format ASCII. Often, when you import data, you find that it contains lots of extra spaces in odd places. A 'stripping' macro can remove all of these extra spaces. Also, if you learned to type on a typewriter, you are probably used to inserting an extra space between sentences. This is not necessary with a wordprocessor and can make a mess of the formatting process. However, I know from experience that this is an almost impossible habit to break. Again, the 'stripping' macro can be run just before you print out your document and it will take out all the extra spaces. The macro is not particularly easy to write but it is worth the time invested in working on it.

These are just a selection of some of the macros that are useful in wordprocessing. All of them mean that the functions listed here can be called up simply by pressing the ALT key and a letter. For example, ALT+B calls up my bullet list macro. Only make macros as the need arises. If you make a whole range of macros at one sitting, you are likely to forget what they do and where they are!

- Make full use of multiple windows. You can usually have many documents or document windows open at any given time. You may, for example, work on your document in one, make notes in another and keep your bibliographical references in a third. Do not, however, be tempted to have the same document open in a variety of windows. This will confuse you when editing and there is no guarantee that you will be able to save all the changes you make to the various versions of the same document.

- Keep your layout simple. Windows wordprocessors make it easy to get carried away with font types, font sizes and complicated layouts. As a rule, stick to a maximum of two font types and four font sizes in any given document. For 'body' text, Times Roman is a good choice and is easy to read. For larger headings, consider a sans serif font such as Helvetica. Avoid fancy fonts altogether unless you are composing an advertisement or a particularly striking visual aid.

- As always, back up your work very frequently.
- If you are new to Windows wordprocessing, make the change slowly. Keep your DOS-based program for working on major projects and use the Windows one for short, new projects. It takes a little while to get used to the new way of working and you need to develop a new mind set.

Example software: **Oxford Writer's Shelf (Oxford University Press)**

Most people who write need to refer to a dictionary fairly frequently. This is a very powerful utility program that every writer will be able to use. It incorporates a number of Oxford University Press dictionaries and reference texts in a simple-to-use program:

- *The Oxford Dictionary for Writers and Editors*
- *The Oxford Minidictionary*
- *The Oxford Miniguide to English Usage*
- *The Oxford Minidictionary of Quotations*

It is possible to conduct random searches, consult an index, search for specific words and phrases highlighted from your documents, and import extracts from texts into your documents. The program works alongside wordprocessors such as WordPerfect and Word.

Most wordprocessors have spellcheckers and the larger ones have a thesaurus. This program is much more than either of those. It allows you to check a meaning, to identify a useful quote and look up certain conventions of layout and grammar.

WRITING PAPERS, ARTICLES AND REPORTS

All of the principles of good writing apply to writing papers, articles and reports. Essentially, the following points are important:

- 'Brainstorm' your ideas before you start to write. A shareware program called PC Outline (Appendix 3) can be useful in helping you to do this. The process involves jotting down all your ideas, in any order, to enable you to be creative in your planning. You then select the really important issues and prioritize these.
- Develop an outline from your brainstorming.
- Open a file on your wordprocessor and set wide margins to allow you to see all of what you write.
- Write quickly at first and do not worry about editing as you go.
- If necessary, leave gaps for references and put them in later.
- When you edit, remember the two basics: use short sentences and short paragraphs. This applies to any sort of writing.

WRITING BOOKS, DISSERTATIONS AND LARGER PROJECTS

Many health professionals have plenty to say about their work and many more could write books than currently do. Many have to complete dissertations, theses and larger projects. There are various stages to book and larger project writing and the process is far easier if you structure what you do. The paragraphs below refer specifically to writing a book. Many of the principles, however, can be adapted for writing a dissertation, thesis or larger project.

First, you need an idea, then you have to contact a publisher and sell them that idea. The publishers, if they are interested, will ask you to prepare a proposal. Most publishers mean the same sort of thing when they ask you for a proposal – they want a short document which identifies the following things:

- the name of the proposed book;
- the author;
- a rationale for the book;
- the market;
- details about the author;
- comparison with other books in the field;

- contents;
- details of length, date of submission and so on.

Once the publishers have received your proposal, an editor will consider it and send it out to one or more reviewers who will be asked to comment on its commercial viability. These stages can take a few months and you would be wise to sit out this period and not to 'worry' the editor. If all goes well, you will then be sent a contract to write the book. You should look at this carefully, sign it and then send it back. You are then under contract to write the book. The next stage is to write it.

I find it useful to plan the outline of the whole on the computer. Open a subdirectory, named after your book. Within this directory, open new files to correspond to the introduction, chapters and bibliography of your book. Just doing this basic housekeeping will help you to feel that you are on your way. You may also want to head each chapter in a standard way so that, when you come to print out, each chapter heading is in the same font and each heading starts at the same point on the page. Here is an example of a possible subdirectory and files for a book on health care:

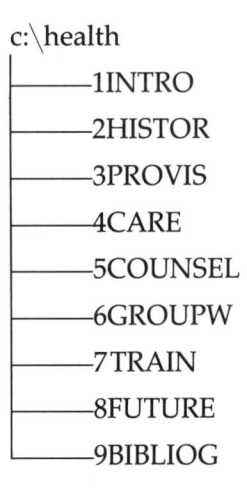

```
c:\health
    ├──1INTRO
    ├──2HISTOR
    ├──3PROVIS
    ├──4CARE
    ├──5COUNSEL
    ├──6GROUPW
    ├──7TRAIN
    ├──8FUTURE
    └──9BIBLIOG
```

The point of using a number at the start of each file name is that this forces each of the files to stay in the order that the chapters appear in the book. This is likely to help you to keep an eye on the length of each chapter in relation to its neighbours and to make accessing files easier.

Don't feel that you have to write a book from cover to cover. The wonderful thing about wordprocessing is that you can write a bit in Chapter 3 and then move to Chapter 6 and then start on Chapter 2. You may find it easier to work on the introduction last of all. By this time, you will have an overall sense of what is in the book and it will help you to discuss the contents and to guide the reader through the book.

Try to discipline yourself as you write. Write a certain number of words every day, if you can, and count the total number of words that you have written each day. This will give you a sense of achievement and allow you to see how you are using your word allowance. Do stick carefully to the word limit. A slim book is usually about 50 000 words in length, a more substantial one might be 70–80 000. If your contract is for 50 000 words, do not write 35 000 or 80 000. It is helpful if you work out the number of words that you can allow yourself for each chapter, before you start writing the book. Try, too, to make the chapters roughly the same length. There is always a temptation to write longer chapters on the topics you know most about.

Write quickly and then edit at leisure. If you find that you hit a 'purple patch' and the words seem to flow easily, work continuously and do not stop to edit – that can come later. It is useful, if you can afford both the paper and the time, to print out a hard copy of your manuscript before you complete the 'final' copy for the publisher. Although this seems to run against the computing grain, there is usually no better way of spotting mistakes and inconsistencies than reading what you have written, from pages rather than from the screen. If you feel that this is too wasteful, make sure that you read the final manuscript through before you send it to the publisher.

Make sure, too, that you have written for permission to use any copyright material in the book. The law is a little blurred in this respect. Under an arrangement called 'fair dealing' you are usually able to quote short passages from other people's publications (as long as you quote the source). If, however, you are at all unsure about whether or not you can make quotes, contact the publishers of the work that you want to use. Most publishers, in my experience, are happy to give such permission and some can be quite generous about their dealings in this respect.

There are certain rules of layout for a manuscript:

- Print on one side of good quality A4 paper but do not use the heaviest of paper. This will merely cost you more money in postage.

- Double space the lines and leave all diagrams and illustrations on separate pages.
- Leave good margins around the edge of your work (about 1½" on all sides).
- Put numbers on all pages and number the manuscript consecutively from the first page to the last. Do not start again at 1 for a new chapter. If you need to insert pages before sending off the manuscript, call the new pages 26b, 26c, etc. If there is a number of extra pages, renumber the entire manuscript. Don't forget that your wordprocessor can automatically number the pages for you. I put the number at the bottom of the page, in the centre. I have read that some publishers prefer page numbers in the top right hand corner.
- Don't use 'headers' or 'footers'. Your aim is not to produce a manuscript that looks like a book but one on which the sub-editor can work. He or she will not thank you if it is necessary to cross out headers and footers on every page.
- Don't use a wide range of fonts. Stick to a standard 10 or 12pt font throughout.
- Do not bind the manuscript at the side. Do not staple it but leave the pages free.
- At the top of each page, print your name and the title of the manuscript. This is just in case anyone drops part of it and then wonders to which pile of papers these particular ones refer. Make sure that you parcel up the manuscript carefully but do not tape it up in such a way that the editor has to fight with the parcel to open it. The boxes that A4 paper are supplied in are often useful for packing two copies of a manuscript.

Example software: Grammatik (Software International)

We all need to improve our writing. Most health care professionals have to write and the ability to do so clearly is an asset. Grammatik, by Software International can help you write even better. The program is grammar checking software that includes writing improvement tools and an extensive spellchecker. One of the best things about it is that it can run within wordprocessors. If, for example, you use WordPerfect, WordStar or Word as your means of getting words into your computer, Grammatik can be popped up to work on the writing that you have just completed. It is not a true 'terminate and stay resident' program but one that works with macros and batch files. It works only with DOS and will not work with Windows, although the company is working on a Windows compatible version.

It would be impossible to list all of Grammatik's functions. Essentially, it is grammar checking software that proofreads wordprocessed documents for errors in grammar, style, usage, punctuation and spelling. It explains errors, gives advice and suggests replacements (where appropriate). It offers a useful means of avoiding jargon, complicated sentences, redundancy and excessive use of the passive voice. In other words, it can help you to write clearer and more lively prose. You can also compare what you have written with different types of styles: general, business, letter, memo, report, technical, journalism and fiction, to name but a few. It also compares your work with a standard business document and (for some reason) one of Churchill's speeches. You can learn a lot from this program. If you are not sure about your grammar, you will be after using Grammatik.

To run the full program through a long document takes time. The program works to so many rules that even a reasonably simple piece is usually taken apart at the seams. This means that the program will stop at every instance of what it considers to be a mistake and offer you the chance to put things right. If you don't like this way of working, you can ask the program to prepare you a special list of mistakes which you can work through later. If you get called away from an editing session, you can use the 'mark' feature to let you come back to where you left off.

As with any style and grammar checker, it has its limitations. It is quite possible to offer it a piece of nonsense written with perfect grammar and spelling. It will assure you that your nonsense is well written and easy to read. The ultimate grammar checker is some way off, but until it arrives Grammatik does the job well.

FURTHER READING

Burnard, P. (1992) *Writing for Health Professionals*, Chapman & Hall, London

In this book, I have tried to describe all the essential processes of writing in the health professions. The book contains chapters on writing essays, projects, educational material and research reports. Many health professionals in colleges and universities have to publish if they are to progress in their careers. In *Writing for Health Professionals* I also describe the process of publishing articles and papers and give hints about how to get into print.

10 Research and the personal computer

Computers can be particularly useful in planning research projects in health care contexts. They can also be invaluable for storing and handling data. This chapter explores practical ways in which the personal computer can be put to use in health care research. It is not intended to be a detailed overview of research methods and data handling but a practical discussion of some of the ways in which computers can help in the research process in the health professions.

PLANNING YOUR RESEARCH PROJECT

All research has to be planned. Using a personal computer can make that planning easier because it can help you to structure your work. These are the headings that you can use for a research proposal:

- **Title.** Keep this short and descriptive.
- **Rationale.** Why do you want to do this research? How does it fit in with what has gone before? This should be about two paragraphs in length and place your research in context.
- **Aims.** Write about three research aims. Only use a hypothesis if you are using an experimental design. Only use an experimental design if you really know what you are doing. Take advice.
- **Sample.** How will you select out respondents from a total population? In the social sciences, it is rare to be able to contact a random sample. In a descriptive, qualitative study, numbers are not so important as the quality of the responses. Be clear about the sampling procedures for both qualitative and quantitative methodologies.

- **Method.** Here you should describe what it is you are going to do. Are you going to do some interviews? Are you going to use a questionnaire? If so, are you going to devise your own questionnaire or will you use someone else's? How will you check for the validity and reliability of your instrument? All of these details should be included in this section of your proposal.
- **Ethical considerations.** Will you have to go before an ethics committee? If so, what preparations have you made? Usually, if you are going to include patients or clients in your sample, you will be required to send your proposal to a local ethics committee. Do make sure that you are clear about your responsibilities in this field.
- **Financial considerations.** How will you pay for the various aspects of your research? Don't forget that you may have a large postage bill if you send out questionnaires. You will also have to pay for paper and for binding the final report. Don't assume that your college will pay for these things.
- **A short CV.** Write a two page curriculum vitae in which you spell out your own background in terms of education, jobs, publications and so forth. The aim of the CV in this case is to support your proposal and to show that you have the relevant experience to complete the research that you have in mind.
- **Timetable.** Write out a plan of action. The 'rule of thirds' is sometimes useful here. One third of your research time should be devoted to searching the literature. Another third will be taken up with data collection and analysis. The final third will see you writing your research report. On the other hand, it is also good practice to write up your work as you go.

Take time preparing the proposal and then print it. As with the book project described in the previous chapter, it is possible to use the chapter headings (in an abbreviated form) as the names of files. You can then set up a directory on your hard disk which contains a file for each of the sections of the research project.

DATA COLLECTION

At least two sorts of research data can be stored in a personal computer: numerical and textual. Numerical data from questionnaires and other forms of survey can be collected in one of two ways: typed directly into a spreadsheet or statistical program, or put into a simple ASCII format so that it can be analysed by a statistical program at a later date. The format for entering data into a spreadsheet is described in Chapter 7. The format for typing data in ASCII format is illustrated in Figure 10.1.

In this example, the first three numbers are 'identifiers': they tell you and the program which respondent (or subject) is being referred to. Then, every figure after this identifier represents a piece of data that can be linked to a codebook. A codebook (which is not necessarily a book at all) is the key to the dataset. It is an essential means of knowing what all the items in a dataset refer to. Data presented in columns and rows, as in Figure 10.1, is called raw data and should never be written into a research report. Such raw data needs, first, to be analysed. Here is an example of a codebook for the data in Figure 10.1.

Columns: 1–3: Respondent identifier

Column: 4 : Gender: 1 = Female, 2 = Male,

Column: 5 : Job: 1 = Social worker, 2 = Doctor, 3 = Nurse

Column: 6 : Question one: All social workers should be trained as AIDS counsellors: 1 = agree, 2 = don't know, 3 = disagree

Column: 7 : Question two: AIDS counselling is a specialist type of counselling: 1 = agree, 2 = don't know, 3 = disagree

Column: 8 : Question three: Most social workers are also 'natural' counsellors: 1 = agree, 2 = don't know, 3 = disagree

Column: 9 : Question four: The most important skill in counselling is listening: 1 = agree, 2 = don't know, 3 = disagree

Column: 10 : Question five: Women tend to make better counsellors than men: 1 = agree, 2 = don't know, 3 = disagree

It should be clear from this example that it would be quite easy to determine, from this dataset, how many doctors agreed with question three, how many social workers disagreed with question four and so on. This is a simple example of frequency counting.

Another sort of data that can be stored in a computer is textual data. This includes everything that is said during an interview. The first stage of working with interview data is to make a full transcription – typing

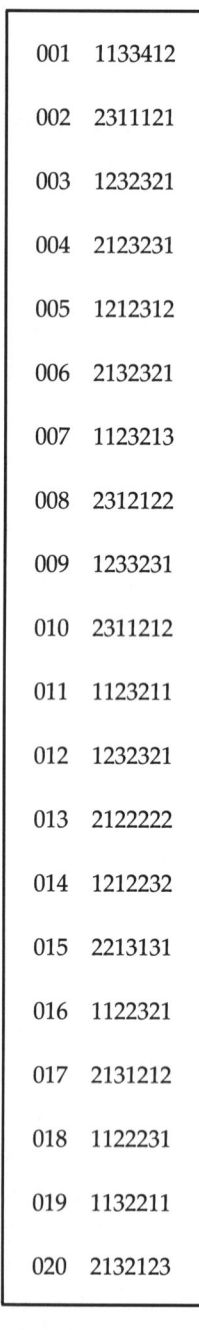

001	1133412
002	2311121
003	1232321
004	2123231
005	1212312
006	2132321
007	1123213
008	2312122
009	1233231
010	2311212
011	1123211
012	1232321
013	2122222
014	1212232
015	2213131
016	1122321
017	2131212
018	1122231
019	1132211
020	2132123

Figure 10.1 Example of an extract from an ASCII dataset.

> **Researcher:** What are you feelings about working with disabled people?
> **Respondent:** I feel I'm always being rushed. I suppose that's an odd thing to say, really. What I mean is that because of the shortage of staff, we never get to do all the things we could do. I mean, we just have to do the basics. They say we are supposed to care for people's psychological needs. I don't know how. We just don't have the time.
> I enjoy it, though. I can't imagine doing anything else, really. Well, I might if I was offered a huge salary (laughs). But, you know what I mean...
> **Researcher:** Does everyone feel rushed?
> **Respondent:** Most of us, I think. The senior social worker doesn't always say so, but I think she feels it too. She feels that she has to support us all the time. I suppose it's difficult for her. She can't really say what she really means. At least, not to me, she can't. I wonder if she tells anyone what she really feels about things? I expect she's like us: she suffers in silence.

Figure 10.2 Example of an interview transcript.

into the computer the words that were spoken during the interview and recorded by a tape recorder. Figure 10.2 offers an example of such data. It is important that when such material is transcribed, plenty of room is allowed around the transcripts for the researcher to make notes. Data of this sort can be analysed in various ways including:

- content analysis of words used;
- content analysis of phrases used;
- content analysis of themes;
- phenomenological analysis of meaning.

One final note needs to be made here. The transcription of interviews is very time consuming. A touch-typist working at full speed is likely to take at least three or four hours to transcribe every hour of interviewing.

DATA ANALYSIS

All research data, quantitative or qualitative, needs to be analysed. Whilst the computer is probably of greatest help in analysing quantitative data, it can also be used to categorize and organize unstructured, qualitative material.

Statistical packages

If you do quantitative work, you may want to do statistical analysis. There are a number of statistical packages you can choose from, many of which are extremely powerful. And herein lies a problem. Because such packages can do so many statistical computations, it is tempting to run these programs to do 'everything' – regardless of whether or not you really understand the analysis that you are doing. Make sure that your data satisfies the criteria for undertaking a particular test before you run the program. Don't forget that the program itself is stupid: there is no program that can determine whether or not it **should** analyse your data using a particular test! It will run the test anyway.

Example software: **C-Stat (Cherwell Scientific)**

C-Stat, produced by Cherwell Scientific is a real find in the research world. It is extremely simple to operate and allows you to work with your data quickly and easily. This simplicity is a key feature. You no longer have to spend hours learning to enter data and then how to get the program to do the analysis. Here, there can be no doubt about how data is to be entered and the pull-down menu system takes you straight to the tests you want.

The program comes on one disk and can either be run from the disk or the files can be copied over to a hard disk. When you start the program you are presented with a spreadsheet (or series of rows and columns). You then type your figures into the spreadsheet, call up the menu and choose your statistical test. A comprehensive range of tests is available: comparison by paired-t, t-test, Mann Whitney U, Wilcoxon signed rank, association by regression, Spearman rank order, linear multiple regression, chi-square, Fisher Exact, McNemar/Yates, Anova and Kruskal Wallis. All of these calculations are performed in the computer memory so that no data is transferred out to disk. This speeds up operation and, despite working in memory in this way, the program can handle large data sets of up to 50 000 items. A wide range of simple calculating functions is also supported.

Simple graphing, bar chart and descriptive plotting facilities are available and quickly called up. These are not the glossy features that you find on some other commercial programs but they offer you the chance to explore your data quickly and easily. Data files from other programs can be read easily and data can also be exported into wordprocessing and graphical programs. Blocks of data can also be cut and pasted within the program. It is the ease with which you can manipulate data that makes the program so attractive.

Many health care professionals on courses are required to complete research projects that involve the handling of numerical data. I suspect that the complicated packages that are available to handle such data do little to allay fears many health care professionals have about handling figures. Also, those larger packages often encourage users to run large numbers of statistical tests on data sets that do not meet the criteria for such tests. This neither increases confidence nor does it make you any clearer about how statistics 'work'. C-Stat, because of its simplicity, is likely to help people to spend more time thinking about the appropriateness of the tests and less time on working out how to use the program.

For any health care researcher, a simple program that is easy to use and yet which covers all of the basic tests is a winner. It would be equally at home on a laptop computer as it would be on a desktop. This is more than can be said for most statistical packages which tend to fill up megabytes of hard disk space.

The handbook that accompanies the program is clearly written and easy to follow. It quickly becomes redundant. It is easy to learn the program 'blind', simply by calling it up and experimenting with the pull-down menus.

Example software: **Unistat Statistical Package (University Software)**

Unistat is an extremely powerful and yet easy to use statistical package. Any health care researcher who needs to work with quantitative data will appreciate being able to explore datasets from a variety of statistical perspectives. Unistat offers ease of data entry, exhaustive statistical analysis and graphical representation of findings – all in one package.

The program is copy protected, which means that you can only make so many copies from the original disks before you run into problems. In this program's case, you can install the program three times. After that, if you make any further installations, you have to use the first program disk to start up the program. The program disk becomes what is known as a 'dongle' in the computing trade. Although I can understand the reasons that programmers and companies have for wanting to copy protect their products, few of the larger companies use such protection.

The program itself is impressive. Its functions can be called up either from the pull-down menus or by typing commands. The spreadsheet part of the program is not only for data entry, it can also be used for various types of 'normal' spreadsheet work. In essence, the package offers two programs in one: a particularly well-featured statistical package and a sophisticated spreadsheet program. This being the case, it offers exceptional value for money. It is quite possible to pay far more than the cost of this program for just a spreadsheet program.

It is impossible to list all of the statistical functions of the program in a review of this size. It can offer a wide range of descriptive statistics, including summaries, confidence intervals and frequency distributions. It also does more than 40 parametric and non-parametric tests including, amongst others, one sample, separate and two sample chi-squared and Kolmogorov-Smirnof tests, Mann Whitney U, Wilcoxon signed rank, Walsh, Wald-Wolfowitz and so on. It also offers Pearson, Spearman and Kendall rank correlations and can generate contingency tables and cross-tabulations. I have never seen a program that offers so many statistical tests and it contains many that I had not come across before. An optional module is available which does cluster analysis, discriminant analysis, multidimensional scaling, principal component analysis, factor analysis and canonical correlations.

The manual is extremely comprehensive. It offers a brief description of the criteria for each of the tests but is not always as clear as it could be. I suspect that this may be due to the fact that the programmer has written the manual. What is clear to a statistician and programmer is not always so clear to a more general reader. Overall, though, this is probably the most comprehensive and easy to use statistical package available at the present time. It is available in both DOS and Windows formats.

Example software: **Survey (Shareware)**

Survey is a simple but extremely useful program that does one task very well. It accepts numerical data from questionnaires and then runs frequency counts for each questionnaire item. Doing multiple frequency counts is something that other programs do not always cope with very easily. Unistat, described above, for example, has problems with it. With Survey, you simply tell the program how many questionnaire items you have and how many variables there are with each item. You then type in the values from your dataset and the program presents you with a series of read-outs for each question. It works best with questionnaires that have Likert-type questions such as the following:

4. Social workers should receive training in AIDS counselling.

Strongly agree	Agree	Don't know	Disagree	Strongly disagree	Leave blank

Survey allows you to quickly identify how many people in a survey answered 'strongly agree', 'agree', 'don't know', disagree' and 'strongly disagree' to this and every other item in the questionnaire.

Qualitative analysis

Not all data is quantitative and not all of it needs to be analysed with a computer. Qualitative data can sometimes be better analysed by hand. If you have detailed transcripts of interviews, for example, you may find it easier to work through the pages and cut and paste as you go. There are, however, computer programs which can help you to analyse qualitative data: the Ethnograph is an example of a giant 'cut and paste' program which is very useful for helping to categorize and organize unstructured data. Wordprocessors such as WordPerfect and Word can also be useful in this respect.

A simple shareware program called WORDFREQ is also useful for doing a content analysis of words in any qualitative data. WORDFREQ presents you with a listing of how many times each word in a document occurs. If you exclude grammatical words such as 'the', this', 'when' and so forth, you can quickly identify the sorts of words that people have been using in interviews.

One method of qualitative data analysis by computer can be described. I used the application described here in a recent research project which reviewed aspects of AIDS counselling (Burnard, 1992). The database program used in this case was Memory Mate (described in Chapter 6).

Memory Mate was used as a tool for content analysis of interview data. Here, the interviews are transcribed and entered into the database as single 'items'. The transcripts can be readily prepared in any word-processor and transferred to the database in the form of ASCII files.

Once the transcripts are in the database, the researcher decides on the categories that he or she wants to use to describe what has been talked about in the interviews. There is not space in this chapter to describe how this can be done but any book about analysing qualitative data can help here.

Supposing, for the moment, that the project is about social workers and AIDS counselling. It is decided that the set of category labels that cover everything that has been discussed in all of the interviews is as follows:

- feelings about AIDS;
- knowledge of AIDS;
- counselling skills;
- counselling courses;
- social workers and the AIDS field;
- caring for people with AIDS;
- AIDS counselling;
- training courses.

The aim is to ensure that any such category system is exhaustive: that everything that any respondent has said in an interview fits into one or other of these category headings.

Next, each of those categories is ascribed an identifying set of letters. For reasons we will see in a moment, it is useful to use rather unusual identifiers. Here is an example:

Data analysis 173

> AAA 'I don't know all that much about it...I suppose I ought to know more.
> I trained some time ago and we didn't have anything on AIDS then...'
>
> BBB 'I need to find out about it. I read something recently – not anything academic, it was an article in a magazine. Still, it was a start...'
>
> CCC 'The article talked about counselling – not AIDS counselling, particularly – about what counsellors do: the skills they are supposed to have, you know. I suppose we all have counselling skills, as social workers. At least, I hope we do. It's difficult, really.'
>
> **KEY:**
>
> AAA Feelings about AIDS
> BBB Knowledge of AIDS
> CCC Counselling skills

Figure 10.3 Example of freeform database text, marked with category codes.

- AAA: Feelings about AIDS;
- BBB: Knowledge of AIDS;
- CCC: Counselling skills;
  and so on.

Once these identifiers have been decided upon, the researcher combs through all of the interviews and marks pieces of text with these identifiers. This is illustrated in Figure 10.3. Once all of the transcripts have been marked up in this way, the researcher simply searches the database for all of the 'AAAs', then all the 'BBBs' and so on. He or she thus brings together all the pieces of the interviews which refer to a particular theme. The reason for using slightly unusual collections of letters is that if these are used, the 'search' mechanism of the program will only stop at the 'AAAs' and the 'BBBs'. If a single 'A' or a single 'B' is used, the search will stop at all examples of the letter 'A'! As can be imagined, this will not be particularly helpful.

WRITING THE REPORT

A research report will strongly echo a research proposal. Most such reports will contain the following chapters:

- Abstract. A short statement of less than 200 words summarizing what your research is about. Use these words carefully. The abstract is all that many people will read of your work. It will appear in abstracting journals and on research databases if it is a study that is being submitted for a Masters degree or PhD. Write the abstract after you have completed your work.
- Acknowledgements. Record your thanks to your supervisor and to your family.
- Introduction. This is a short chapter which offers an overview of what is to come.
- Chapter One: Literature review;
- Chapter Two: Aims of the study;
- Chapter Three: Methodology;
- Chapter Four: Analysis;
- Chapter Five: Findings;
- Chapter Six: Discussion of Findings;
- Chapter Seven: Conclusions;
- Chapter Eight: Applications and Limitations;
- References;
- Appendices.

It is not usual to index your research report although this may become a standard feature as more people work with wordprocessors. Avoid too many appendices: they can appear to be page-filling and often are. Also avoid a bibliography unless your funding authority or tutor has asked for one. The difference between a reference list and a bibliography is this. A reference list is a listing of all of the works that you have referred to, directly, in your research. A bibliography is a separate listing of other books that are related to the topic but which are not referred to in your work. In practice, bibliographies are very easy to compile, especially with the use of CD-ROM and other searching facilities. Bibliographies which are compiled in this way are merely a list of books and articles that the researcher has managed to find on the particular topic. Generally, it is better to stick to a reference list only.

FURTHER READING

Sommer, B. and Sommer, R. (1991) *A Practical Guide to Behavioural Research: Tools and Techniques*, 3rd edn, Oxford University Press, Oxford

Not specifically a computing book but an excellent and clearly written introduction to the process of doing research in the social sciences. Not particularly strong on qualitative methods, this book offers lots of straightforward advice (including computing advice) about how to do research. I think it is one of the best introductory texts on research methods there is.

References

Baker, J. (1987) *Copy Prep*, Blueprint, London.
Bray, P. (1992) What's in a floppy? *PC Direct*, July, 380–4.
Budgett, H. (1992) The PC Direct guide to buying DTP software. *PC Direct*, July, 412–16.
Burnard, P. (1992) *Perceptions of AIDS Counselling*, Avebury, Aldershot.
Gunning, R. (1968) *The Techniques of Clear Writing*, 2nd edn, McGraw Hill, London.
Jones, S. (1992) Making the upgrade. *PC Direct*, July, 422–8.
Monteith, M. (1992) Writing: a historical perspective, in *Teaching Creative Writing* (eds M. Monteith and R. Miles), Open University Press, Milton Keynes.
Peckitt, R. (1989) *Computers in General Practice*, Sigma Press, Wilmslow.
Pfaffenberger, B. (1991) *Que's Computer User's Dictionary*, Que Corporation, Carmel, Indiana.
Waddilove, R. (1992) Making the move. *PC Today*, **6**(2), 181–2.

Appendix 1
Glossary of computer terms[1]

Adaptor Normally refers to the circuit, usually in the form of an expansion card, that connects to the monitor to generate the video display. See *MDA, Hercules, CGA, EGA, VGA, SVGA*.

Application A program or collection of programs that makes the PC carry out a specific job such as being a wordprocessor or a database system.

ASCII American Standard Code for Information Interchange. Usually pronounced 'askey'. Computers only deal with numbers (see *byte* and *bit*) so each character of text must be represented by a numeric code. Capital A is 65, B is 66 and so on. ASCII is a widely used list specifying which numbers represent which characters.

Assembler A language where the programmer is working directly with the CPU. Long-winded and hard to write, but the only way to extract maximum performance when it matters. Other languages trade off ease of use for slower execution speed and larger program files. See *machine code*.

AT Advanced technology. An IBM model designation for its first PC with an 80286 CPU. Now often applied to machines with 80386 and i486 CPUs.

Back up The process of copying data from one storage medium, for instance a hard disk, to another such as floppy disks or a tape streamer. The back-up copy can be used if the original is accidentally destroyed.

BASIC Beginner's All-purpose Symbolic Instruction Code. One of the easiest languages for writing programs. Many PCs come supplied with a version of BASIC.

---

[1] Reproduced with permission from *PC Answers*, Future Publishing Ltd, Bath, Avon

Benchmark A test of the performance (usually speed) of a piece of software or hardware. In the case of hardware, a special benchmark program runs the tests and displays the results.

Bernoulli drive A type of disk drive that uses large removable cartridges up to 90Mb capacity. The name derives from a phenomenon known as the Bernoulli effect. It concerns the way the edge of a spinning flexible disk is sucked towards, but never touches, a stationary surface. In the drive this is arranged so that the disk gets sucked from a sagging position into a horizontal one. The read/write head pokes through the surface.

Binary Numbers written in base 2 where a digit can only be 0 or 1. Decimal 1, 2, 3, 4, 5 translate as 1, 10, 11, 100, 101. See *byte* and *bit*.

BIOS Usually refers to programs permanently recorded in a chip (a read-only memory, or ROM) fitted to the PC. DOS and applications can use them to perform basic input and output operations like screen printing, hence the name Basic Input/Output System.

Bit A byte is divided into eight bits. Each bit can represent the digits 1 or 0. Eight digits in binary notation can form numbers whose decimal values are between 0 and 255. In a memory chip, a bit is really a tiny electronic switch that can only be either on or off.

Boot The process the PC goes through when it starts up – it checks itself, then loads the operating system from disk. 'Re-boot' means to force the PC to go through its start-up sequence again.

BubbleJet Canon's proprietary name for its ink jet printers.

Bus A circuit that carries data between different parts of the computer: the data transport equivalent of a motorway.

Byte A unit of storage capacity in a computer: a memory cell. It will hold a number between 0 and 255. These numbers can be used as codes to represent text characters: see *ASCII*. They can also represent instructions to the CPU. See *bit* and *machine code*.

C A powerful and not particularly easy language.

Cache (disk) An area of memory used to store a copy of data recently read from or written to a hard disk. When a program requests data from the disk, if it is in the cache it can be supplied a lot more quickly than bringing the disk mechanism into play. The result is to speed up operation of the program. The more memory allocated to the cache, the more chance there is of the required data being in there. A disk cache is usually set up by a special utility. See *memory cache*.

CAD Computer aided design or computer assisted drafting, depending on who you listen to. An application program that turns the PC into the equivalent of a draughtsman's drawing board and instruments. See *pen plotter*.

CD-ROM Compact Disk Read-Only Memory. Like an audio CD but used as a storage medium for programs and data. Very high capacity but the PC cannot save information on it, only read from it. Used to distribute a large quantity of material that doesn't need to be changed.

Cell See *spreadsheet*.

Centronics See *parallel port*.

CGA Colour graphics adaptor – IBM's first attempt at a colour display adaptor. Chunky characters and graphics coupled with limited colours make it seem crude by today's standards. See *MDA, EGA*.

Character A letter, numeral, punctuation mark or special symbol that can be displayed on the screen or printer. See *ASCII*.

Chip A complex electronic circuit formed in a one-piece silicon wafer. It is housed in a thin rectangular block (usually black) with external metal contacts. Often known as an integrated circuit (IC) which originally meant miniaturized conventional components on a circuit board housed in a larger package.

Clone A PC not made by IBM but which will run the same software and use the same hardware add-ons as a genuine IBM machine.

CMOS Complementary metal oxide semiconductor. Used to make chips that need to run with low power requirements. The CMOS RAM in an AT-class machine is a small area of battery powered memory used to store certain settings while the PC is switched off, such as the type of hard disk fitted and the current time.

Colour palettes The PC can only display a finite number of colours on the screen at any one time, the exact number depending on the video adaptor you have fitted. For example, in some cases only 16 colours may be permitted. Some adaptors have the facility to choose each colour from a wider selection called the palette, so it might be a case of any 16 from a palette of 64. However, the term 'palette' is sometimes applied to the 16 colours rather than the 64, so you have to look at the context to decide exactly what is meant.

Comms Short for communications. The act of exchanging data between computers, often via the telephone system using a modem.

Controller In the context of disks, means an electronic circuit that acts as an interface between the software and the drive. Programs needing to read from or write to the disk say what they want, and the controller is responsible for operating the mechanism.

CPU Central processing unit: the chip with ultimate control of your PC. It is told what to do by programs. The CPU chips used in PCs were designed by Intel and given an identifying number: 8088, 8086, 80286, 80386 and i486, in increasing order of power and capability. See also *V20/V30* and *SX* chips.

Crash A serious program malfunction which has unpredictable results. Often the PC locks up entirely, and you have to re-boot.

Daisywheel A printer where characters are formed by a technique similar to that used by typewriters. A set of hammers (known as petals) is mounted radially on a wheel, the daisywheel or printwheel, which is rotated to bring the correct one into line. Daisywheel printers are incapable of reproducing graphics.

Data Information in a computer system being processed by a program, for example, names in a database or figures in a spreadsheet. Confusingly, the data being processed may be another program, for instance in the context of a disk cache, 'data' may include program files.

Database A program that stores information, for example a list of names and addresses or a book catalogue, in such a way that it can easily be retrieved by use of searching and sorting facilities. The information is typically stored in records, each record corresponding to a card in a conventional index. Within each record are one or more fields. If the database contained a list of names and addresses, for example, each person would have their own record within which their name, the lines of their address, and the telephone number would have their own fields.

Default When something must be specified, for example when an installation program asks you to name the hard disk directory into which it will copy files from a floppy disk, the default is a setting used if you choose not to specify something of your own.

Digitizer pad A pad and input device which either looks like a mouse with an integral cross-hair or a stylus. It is used for accurate positioning of an on-screen pointer. The stylus or mouse-like component (puck) is used in conjunction with the special pad, allowing software to determine its location in relation to a coordinate system. This contrasts with a mouse where only its motion relative to its last position can be determined.

Glossary of Computer Terms

Dingbat See *Zapf Dingbats*

DIP Dual in-line package, a chip where the connectors form two lines, one down each long side.

Disk General term covering various types of media used to permanently store program and data files. In most cases they can be both read from and written to by the PC. See *drive, hard disk, floppy disk* and *CD-ROM*. Many types (though not all of them: see *optical drive*) rely on a magnetic coating similar to that employed on audio tapes. Before information can be saved on such a disk, it must be recorded with a pattern of concentric rings (tracks) which are subdivided into sectors. See *format*.

Dos Disk operating system. Also see *MS-DOS* and *DR-DOS*.

Dot matrix A printer where the characters and graphics are formed from a grid of dots (matrix) produced by wire pins.

DR-DOS Digital Research disk operating system. A competitor to MS-DOS that will run the same software and obey the same or similar commands.

Drive In the context of a disk, the mechanism that holds the storage medium and reads and writes the information.

DTP Desktop publishing. An application program for designing pages of graphics and text as found in magazines, newsletters, adverts and the like.

EGA Enhanced graphics adaptor. A step up from CGA offering a sharper image by virtue of there being more dots on the screen, plus more colours. Also see *VGA*.

EISA Extended industry standard architecture. A non-IBM design of PC more advanced than AT and XT machines. It is a competitor to MCA. Also see *ISA*.

E Mail An electronic postal system that stores messages on a central computer, usually in the form of text files, although programs and other data can be handled too. Messages are sent via a PC and a modem link or network.

EMS See *expanded memory*.

Expanded/extended memory Different ways of adding memory beyond the basic 640k. Expanded memory (also known as LIM EMS – Lotus Intel Microsoft Expanded Memory Specification) can be fitted to all PCs. Hardware restrictions dictate that it works differently from normal memory, and programs have to be specially designed to use it. Expanded memory acts like a notebook which applications can employ for additional data storage capacity. Design limitations in the 8088 and 8086 CPU chips mean that PCs fitted with them cannot have extended memory: you need an 80286 or better. Extended memory simply adds more RAM on top of the bottom 1024k normally supplied with these PCs. Unfortunately MS-DOS and most programs run from it cannot normally use extended memory, or at least do so in a very limited way. However, some products such as Windows 3 can take full advantage of it. Extended memory can also be made to mimic expanded RAM if that's the only type your software will work with.

Expansion card A circuit board that fits into an expansion slot.

Expansion slot A socket inside the PC into which can be plugged circuit boards that add extra capabilities to the machine.

FDD Floppy disk drive.

Field See *database*.

File A self-contained body of information stored on disk that can be retrieved at a later date. It can be a program, a document from a wordprocessor, an address list from a database, a year's sales figures from a spreadsheet or whatever. The file is given a name, the filename, so that you can refer to it.

Floppy disk A flexible disk, although it may be contained in a rigid case, that is removable from the drive. Two sizes are available for the PC: 5¼" and 3½". Each size comes in two or more capacities. Floppies have less storage space, are slower and, in the long run, less reliable than other types of disk.

Font Strictly speaking, a particular size and style of a typeface, for example 14pt Times Italic. Times is the design (the typeface), Italic is its style (slanted), and 14pt (14 point) is a measure of the height of the characters. In computing, the term 'font' is often used to mean typeface.

Format Used mainly in two contexts. To format a disk means to lay down a structure of tracks and sectors ready to receive programs and data. A file format is a set of rules governing the way information is structured inside a file. Any program that knows the rules can read or write files that conform to them. For example, graphics files are often in a format known as PCX. In theory, a painting, DTP or wordprocessor program that understands the rules governing PCX can make sense of PCX files produced by other software.

Graphics Any screen or hard copy output where pictures are constructed from tiny dots allowing virtually anything to be drawn. See *MDA* and *Hercules*.

Hard disk A combined disk and drive mechanism usually permanently fixed inside the PC, but removable and portable external versions exist. Much faster and far higher capacity than a floppy disk, so they are frequently used for primary day-to-day storage.

Hardware The electronics and mechanical units that go together to make up the computer and its peripherals.

HDD Hard disk drive.

Hercules A company which produces a mono display adaptor combining MDA-standard text-only output with a special graphics mode. Hercules produces other products, including top-end colour adaptors, but its name is often used to refer to this old widely adopted mono standard.

Hexadecimal Often shortened to 'hex' and meaning numbers in base 16. Decimal (base 10) numbers 1–15 are represented as 1, 2, 3, 4, 5, 6, 7, 8, 9, A, B, C, D, E, F. Decimal 16 becomes hexadecimal 10, and so on. Mainly of interest to programmers.

IBM International Business Machines: the company that designed the original PC and is still a leading manufacturer. See also *clone*.

IC Integrated circuit: see *chip*.

IDE Integrated drive electronics. Refers to a hard disk drive where much of the circuitry that used to be on the hard disk controller card is fitted to the drive unit. See also *interface*.

Ink-jet A printer where characters and graphics are formed from a grid of dots (a matrix) produced by fine ink nozzles. See *BubbleJet*.

Interface Software or hardware that sits between two other pieces of software or hardware and acts as a go-between. Without the interface they cannot communicate with each other. An example would be a hard disk controller which allows the PC to control the mechanism to save and retrieve files.

Interleave factor Usually mentioned in connection with hard disks. It describes one aspect of the way information is arranged on the disk. The lower the ratio stated, the faster data can be transferred, with 1:1 being the optimum.

ISA Industry standard architecture: the design of PC usually classed as an AT. See *EISA* and *MCA*.

k Kilobyte (1024 bytes).

LAN Local area network. A network on one site where all devices on the network are directly connected together. Also see *WAN*.

Language A way of writing programs. Different languages have different ways of telling the PC what to do, some being better than others for particular types of tasks. DOS and all your .EXE and .COM files were written with a language. See *machine code*.

Laser printer A printer which uses photocopier technology to output high-quality pages of text and graphics.

LIM EMS See *expanded memory*.

Machine code Numeric instruction codes understood by the CPU. Languages except assembler generate several machine code instructions for each command. In assembler, one command translates to one instruction.

Macro A stored sequence of keystrokes that can be replayed by pressing just one or two keys or by entering a short command. It's a short-cut to save typing.

Mail merge The process whereby, for example, multiple copies of a letter created with a wordprocessor can have names and addresses read in from a database and inserted at designated points to form personalized correspondence.

Maths coprocessor A chip inside a PC that speeds up programs which do a lot of calculations using floating point numbers: numbers with a fractional part. Programs must be specially written to take advantage of the chip if it is fitted. Common maths coprocessors can be numbered 8087, 80287, 80387SX, 80387DX or i487SX depending on the type of CPU they are designed to work with. The i486DX has a coprocessor built in, but the i486SX does not.

Mb Megabyte (1024k, therefore 1 048 576 bytes).

MCA Microchannel architecture. IBM's latest design of PC that it would like to supersede machines based on the XT and AT standards. See *EISA*.

MDA Mono display adaptor. IBM's original screen display standard. It could only generate text, and so was unsuitable for the construction of pictures from individual dots. See *Hercules* and *CGA*.

Memory Electronic circuits that store programs and data when they are active. See *RAM* and *ROM*. Not to be confused with the hard disk.

Memory cache A small area of fast memory (it can be written to or read from quicker than most memory chips) separate from the PC's main memory pool. It is used to store the most frequently accessed sections of the currently running program. Consequently they run more quickly and the program speeds up. Fast memory tends to be expensive, hence its use in a cache rather than for all the RAM in the machine. See *disk cache*.

MFM Modified frequency modulation: a common method of storing information on the surface of a hard disk. See *RLL*.

MIDI Musical instrument digital interface. A standard connector and communications technique that allows suitably equipped computers and musical instruments to control each other to greatly expand their musical processing abilities.

Modem *M*odulator/*dem*odulator: a hardware device that connects to the PC and allows it to communicate worldwide with other computers via the telephone system. See *comms*.

Mouse A device that can be pushed around your desk to control an on-screen pointer. At least two buttons are used to select menu items and perform actions on objects. Connects either to a serial port or mouse socket. See *WIMP*.

MS-DOS Microsoft disk operating system. See *operating system*.

Multimedia Using the PC to blend motion and still video, hi-fi sound, computer generated text and graphics to present information such as a training course or a catalogue of animals in an interactive way.

Multitasking Running more than one program or doing more than one job simultaneously.

Network A way of linking several PCs together so that they can swap files and share resources such as printers and hard disks. Printing across a network means outputting to a printer on the network rather than one attached to your own printer port. Also see *LAN* and *WAN*.

Operating system A program which is automatically loaded into your PC when it is switched on and provides the A>, B> or C> prompt. When you type a command it either acts on it if it is built in – COPY, for example – or looks for a program of that name on the disk and runs it.

Optical drive A form of disk drive that involves the use of laser light as part of the recording/retrieval process. There are several competing types, not all of which are commercially available. Some drives mix magnetic and optical techniques, and may be referred to as magneto-optical drives.

OS/2 An operating system devised by IBM and Microsoft, intended as the successor to MS-DOS. It does, however, have rivals and its ultimate success is not yet clear. Microsoft recently pulled out, leaving development of OS/2 in the hands of IBM.

Parallel port A socket on the back of your PC that can be used to exchange information with other devices that also have a parallel port fitted. It is usually used with a printer and often known as a Centronics port. It employs a faster technique than that used by the *serial port*.

Pascal A language – used a lot in education – that is powerful enough to be used in commercial programming projects.

PC The IBM Personal Computer, its clones and successors.

PCW A non-PC computer made by Amstrad. It is mainly used for wordprocessing.

PCX A graphics file format.

Pen plotter Akin to a printer, but works by moving pens over the surface of the paper. Often used in conjunction with CAD software to produce engineering drawings, for example.

Peripheral Strictly speaking, any device connected to the core computing circuitry of CPU and memory, for example the disk drives. Often taken to mean items outside the case, such as printers.

Pixel Each dot (*pic*ture *el*ement) on the screen.

Plotter See *pen plotter*.

Portable PC A small PC designed to be carried around. Some models have batteries so they can be used on the move.

PostScript A type of computer programming language which is understood by some laser printers. Commands in PostScript do such things as print text, draw lines and fill areas. A PostScript file is a complete set of instructions that tells the printer how to draw one or more pages.

Printer A piece of hardware that the PC uses to print text and graphics on paper. See *daisywheel*, *dot matrix*, *ink jet* and *laser*.

Program A sequence of numeric instruction codes that tell the CPU what to do. Since the CPU controls the rest of the machine, a program can access all the available facilities: memory, screen, keyboard, mouse, disk drives and so on. By executing programs the PC's hardware is made to act as a wordprocessor, spreadsheet, database or whatever. A programmer is either a person who writes programs, or a device for putting programs into ROMs.

RAM Random access memory: these are the circuits that store a program loaded from disk while it is being executed by the CPU.

RAM is also used by the program as a storage area for its data. When the power is removed from RAM, its contents are lost. See *ROM*.

Re-boot See *boot*.

Record See *database*.

Resolution A computer display is composed of rows and columns of dots from which all characters, lines and filled areas are built. Resolution is a measure of the number of rows and columns. On the screen, for example, 320 × 256 means 320 dots across and 256 high. Printers measure resolution slightly differently. Instead of the total number of dots, it is the number of dots per inch, or dpi. The more dots in an area, the higher the resolution and the crisper the display.

RLL Run length limited: a method of storing information on a hard disk in which data is compressed, compared to MFM, to give around 50% extra capacity and faster data transfer rate.

ROM Read-only memory. Cannot be written to by the CPU but it does not lose data when the power is switched off. Used by hardware manufacturers to incorporate programs and data that must be permanently available. Also see *RAM*.

RS232 The name of an international standard governing the way a serial port works. RS232 is often used instead of 'serial port'.

Scanner A device which scans photographs or other illustrations to create either greyscale or colour images for use in a DTP program, for example.

SCSI Small computer systems interface. A general purpose high-speed multitasking electronic interface used to connect a computer to peripheral devices such as suitably equipped printers and disk drives. Up to seven devices can be joined to one SCSI port.

Sector See *disk*.

Serial port A socket on the back of your PC that can be used to connect it to a computer or other device such as a mouse, modem or pen plotter that also has a serial port. It is used to send and receive information. Also known as RS232. See *parallel port*.

SIM/SIMM Single in-line memory module – very like an SIP except there are no legs. Instead there are metal strips on the edge of the device which fit into a socket. See also *DIP*.

SIP Single in-line package: a chip or set of chips mounted on a miniature circuit board, with connector legs in one line along an edge. See *SIM* and *DIP*.

Software Programs and data stored in the computer or on media such as disks.

Spreadsheet A program used to store and perform calculations on figures. It is based on a grid of cells corresponding to the squares on a piece of ruled paper. Each cell can contain explanatory text, a number, or a formula that acts upon the contents of other cells.

SVGA Super video graphics array: VGA with extra facilities worth having if your software supports them. Not an IBM standard, but one devised by third-party video adaptor manufacturers. See *VGA* and *XGA*.

SX chips The 386SX is a version of the 386 CPU. It does almost everything a 386 (or 80386DX, to give it its full name) can do, but fits circuit boards using components intended to work with the older 80286 CPU. The result is a cheaper PC which has a 386 PC's special capabilities but runs slower. The 486SX is a version of the 486 CPU (now known as the i486DX). It lacks the 486's on-board maths coprocessor, but retains other improvements of the 486 over the 386. A 487SX maths coprocessor is available.

Tape streamer A device used to keep a copy of files from a hard disk. These back-up files are stored on a tape cartridge which is removed and kept somewhere safe. In the event of files being accidentally lost from the hard drive, they can easily be restored.

Toner Powder pigment used by laser printers to make an image on paper or overhead projector film.

Toolkit Applicable to specialist areas such as programmers' toolkits, but in general means a collection of programs that perform maintenance, repair and other routine tasks. For example, a toolkit may be able to revive deleted files, fix corrupted disks and make disk copying easier. The list of functions varies from one package to another.

Track See *disk*.

Tracker ball Rather like a mouse on its back: the device remains stationary and you rotate the ball to move an on-screen pointer.

TSR Terminate and stay resident: a program designed to remain quickly accessible even while another application is running, often by pressing a special key combination known as the hot key. A TSR can stop being active (Terminate) but still remain in the PC's RAM (Stay Resident).

Typeface See *font*.

Glossary of Computer Terms

V20/V30 CPU chips made by NEC. Equivalent to Intel's 8088/8086 chips but work up to 30% faster.

VGA Video graphics array. IBM's third stab at a mass-market colour video adaptor. Still more colours and higher resolution than EGA. Until recently the most popular standard on new machines, though SVGA has probably overtaken it now.

Virus A program that secretly installs itself in a PC and tampers with the system to ensure it gets run automatically. The virus makes copies of itself and thereby spreads to other PCs, usually via floppy disks. Some viruses have no bad effects while others wipe data from disks or do something else destructive. Because of media hype they are often blamed for trouble they don't cause, though the threat they present demands that suitable precautions be taken to protect against infection.

WAN Wide area network: a network that spreads over several sites. Each site will have a local network system (LAN), and talk to the other systems by means of modem or radio link.

WIMP Acronym for windows, icons, menus, pointer (or windows, icons, mouse, pull-down menus, depending on who you listen to). It's the general name for easy-to-use systems like Windows and GEM where the PC's screen imitates a desktop on which there are folders and pieces of paper. Items are represented graphically and selected by moving the pointer and clicking the mouse button. Actions are invoked from menus pulled down from a bar at the top of the screen. Modern WIMPs rarely have the mouse as the sole means of control, but they are generally easier to use with one.

Winchester Another name (slang) for a hard disk, named after the Winchester 30-30 rifle. An early IBM hard disk was known as the 30-30 drive because it had 30Mb of permanent storage and 30Mb of removable storage.

Wordprocessor A program used instead of a typewriter, with extra features such as the ability to delete text, move blocks of it around the document and check the spelling. Only when you're happy with your work need you put it on paper with a printer.

WYSIWYG Pronounced 'wizzy-wig'. An acronym for 'what you see is what you get'. Refers to programs that accurately represent on the screen the appearance of the final printed output. Most DTP programs as well as a smaller number of wordprocessors are WYSIMYG.

XGA Extended graphics array. IBM's newest video adaptor, intended to supersede VGA, but yet to find its way into the mass clone market. See also *SVGA*.

XT Extra technology: an IBM model designation now generally accepted to mean any PC with an 8088 or 8086 CPU.

Zapf Dingbats A typeface, designed by Hermann Zapf, that is composed of special symbols such as arrows, stars and the like. Also see *font*.

Appendix 2
Examples of commercial software

This appendix offers brief descriptions of some of the commercial programs that are available and that will be of use to a variety of health care professionals. Appendix 3 offers details of some of the shareware programs that are available. The program details in this appendix are reproduced with permission from *Computer Buyer*, a Dennis Publication.

WORDPROCESSING PACKAGES

The features that you need from a wordprocessor will depend on the sort of documents that you're producing. The simplest of packages will be good enough if all you want to do is write a letter to the social worker, but if you are producing documentation or writing a thesis, you may need something more advanced, like different headers and footers on alternate pages. WYSIWYG, or what you see is what you get, means that the screen display will look almost exactly like the printed page. Some of the packages go half way towards this with a preview option. Other useful features for people producing long documents include the ability to link files so that you can save chapters or sections separately but still print them out as one document, to produce tables of contents or create documents from outlines.

DOS applications

Better Working Word (Blueneck Computers)

A surprisingly well featured wordprocessor for the price. Six typefaces are available from 5pt to 60pt. A dictionary, thesaurus and outliner are included.

Appendix 2

Cliqword (Quadratron Systems UK)

Integrates with the other Cliq modules. An add-on package with diary, notepad, address book and E Mail is available.

Displaywrite (IBM UK)

Displaywrite provides an interface that allows other PC applications to access its functions and is also capable of exchanging documents with IBM systems including AS/400 and System 36. Up to three dictionaries can be used.

Format-PC (Elite Software Company)

A straightforward package for people who want to process simple documents. Supports Russian program for the same prices on request. Sophisticated Arabic language is also an option.

Galaxy Pro-Lite (Shareware Marketing)

Galaxy Pro-Lite is an extremely basic wordprocessing package but if all you need is to create simple documents, it may be enough.

LetterPerfect (WordPerfect UK)

LetterPerfect is a cut-down version of WordPerfect, lacking many of the advanced features that make the latter so popular. It also suffers from having a restricted range of file exchange formats.

LEX Elite (Ace Microsystems)

A fully featured wordprocessor, which is also a small-scale integrated package with database and application builder. Also has calculator for ledgers and cost analysis. Imports 1-2-3 files.

LocoScript PC (Locomotive Software)

The PC version of the program originally written for the Amstrad PCW is mainly of interest to those migrating from the PCW. The printer support is not very flexible by modern standards.

Manuscript (Lotus Developments UK)

Manuscript includes support for downloadable fonts and is able to import a wide range of graphics formats, including Macintosh and PostScript files. A licence for the Word-4-Word conversion package is included.

Examples of Commercial Software 195

Multiword (Multisoft Financial Systems)

Designed around the standard Multisoft products, so, for example, it integrates with Multisoft Accounts. Offers full WYSIWYG, line drawing for forms and diagrams, and information retrieval.

PC Scribe (The Sage Group)

Despite the low price, PC Scribe has many features found in relatively sophisticated packages, such as an outlining facility and style sheets. But it also includes less useful features such as a grammar checker.

Protext (Arnor)

Not a particularly intuitive package, though at the price, it is fairly fully featured. You have to invest a certain amount of effort in this package to get the most out of it.

Range Text Manager (Transaction Point)

Oriented towards an ICL based system and can be integrated into ICL's Office Power. A fully featured wordprocessor in its own right.

Samna Word (Lotus Developments UK)

A relatively pricey package distinguished only by its ability to process equations for scientists. Password protection and file locking are included.

SmartWare (Informix Software)

This package is one of the modules of the SmartWare integrated system and is supplied with the Smart comms module and programming language.

Tassword PC (Tasman Software)

Tassword PC has few features but it is a very simple package to use and about the cheapest wordprocessor on the market.

Textor (Computer Associates)

Low priced wordprocessor with pull-down menus, font support and page preview. Up to eight documents can be opened at once.

TopCopy Plus 2 (Toplevel Computing)

TopCopy Plus is a cut-down version of TopCopy Professional. It too can be installed as a pop-up application. The price includes three months of free telephone support.

TopCopy Professional (Toplevel Computing)

This package provides features, such as multiple columns, not found on some expensive programs. It can be used as a memory resident program, making it accessible from other programs.

Volkswriter (Volkswriter UK)

Volkswriter 4 includes the Grammatik grammar checker and is available with a range of 'luxury options' including legal and medical dictionaries.

Vuwriter (Vuman Computer Systems)

This basic wordprocessor has a selection of Russian and Greek fonts as well as a range of European character styles; it also provides a wide range of scientific symbols. It can also handle equations.

Word (Microsoft)

This package is able to exchange files with both Windows and OS/2 versions and can import a wide range of graphics formats. A macro system makes it easy to automate frequently performed command sequences.

Wordcheck Plus (Quest Software)

This package can be used as a stand-alone or integrated with Quest's Checkbook accounts software. It also contains a flat file database.

Wordcraft (Wordcraft International)

Designed for secretaries who are processing large amounts of text, Wordcraft is very fast but not necessarily easy to get to grips with. It has a powerful database for mail shots.

WordPerfect (WordPerfect UK)

One of the most popular wordprocessors, WordPerfect provides all the facilities that most people are likely to need. It is now available for the Macintosh and in various Unix versions, as well as on the PC under DOS and Windows.

WordStar (WordStar International)

Although one of the oldest wordprocessors on the market, WordStar provides a full range of features while still remaining compatible with previous versions.

Write On (Software Production)

A simple but colourful wordprocessor for schoolchildren, this full-colour package can be configured as users become more skilled. It has more typefaces and features such as graphics importing than you might expect for the price.

Windows and graphical applications

Ami Pro (Lotus Developments UK)

This package provides a comprehensive range of tools, a macro language and support for OLE.

JustWrite (Symatec)

A full-featured wordprocessor which automatically recognizes the file formats of several other programs and fully supports Windows DDE (dynamic data exchange) for the inclusion of graphics and other data in your documents.

Lotus Write (Lotus Developments UK)

Cut-down version of the much more expensive Ami Pro, Lotus has stripped out that package's advanced features to come up with this entry level wordprocessor for Windows.

Professional Write (Software Publishing Corporation)

Support for MHS compatible E Mail systems is included in this package, along with Windows DDE for the inclusion of automatically updated information for other programs, and a grammar checker. A wide range of file formats can be read.

Textor for Windows (Computer Associates)

Extensively redesigned version of the DOS wordprocessor, making comprehensive use of Windows. Adds full WYSIWYG and headers and footers, with alternate paragraph numbering.

Word for Windows (Microsoft)

Latest versions of Word for Windows feature drag and drop editing of text. WordPerfect keystrokes are recognized.

WordPerfect for Windows (WordPerfect UK)

This Windows version of WordPerfect is keystroke compatible with the DOS version but provides added functionality such as Windows DDE.

WordStar for Windows (WordStar International)

This package accepts the same keystrokes as the DOS version. Its use of frames for document layout gives it more of a DTP feel than most other wordprocessors.

1st Word Plus (Digital Research)

Provides the graphical capabilities that need much more powerful hardware but lacks some of the features that are necessary for more sophisticated work, such as outlining and multiple columns.

K-Word 2 (Kuma Computers)

Data created with K-Word is compatible with Kuma's other K series products, such as K-Graph, K-Spread and K-Data, so data can be included in reports and presentations.

SPREADSHEETS

Spreadsheets are one of the most flexible applications available; most of them have database functions as well as the more usual mathematical ones. If you perform lots of complex operations, look for a macro system so that you can automate frequently performed tasks. Many of the packages will generate graphs and pie charts from your data. If looks are important, choose a package with WYSIWYG so that you can see what the printouts will look like.

DOS applications

Lotus 1-2-3 (Lotus Developments UK)

One of the most popular spreadsheets available for the PC, this package is flexible and powerful, though its menu structure can be a little confusing at times.

PlanPerfect (WordPerfect UK)

PlanPerfect provides the same background print queuing facilities as WordPerfect and is able to automatically convert a WordPerfect table into spreadsheet information.

Procube 3D (CDL)

This program will handle the usual range of spreadsheet, maths and scientific functions and import and export Lotus 1-2-3, dBase, TIF and ASCII files.

Quattro Pro (Borland)

Quattro Pro is capable of reading files created by Borland's Paradox database.

Quattro Pro SE (Borland)

Quattro Pro Special Edition provides many of the same features of the full-blown package at a fraction of the price, though it lacks WYSIWYG.

SmartWare (Informix Software)

This program is part of the SmartWare II integrated package and is supplied with the Smart programming language and communications module.

SuperCalc (Computer Associates)

SuperCalc provides three-dimensional spreadsheets, a wide range of graphs formats and the ability to work with the same menus as Lotus 1-2-3.

Words and Figures (Volkswriter UK)

This package has an integrated wordprocessor. You can insert an active wordsheet region into the text and Words and Figures instantly updates the spreadsheet to reflect those changes.

Windows and graphical applications

Excel (Microsoft)

Both the Windows and the Macintosh versions of Excel use the same file formats, making use on mixed networks easy. A wide range of graphs can be automaticallygenerated from spreadsheet data.

Wingz for Windows (Informix Software)

Wingz is available on both Macintosh and Unix platforms in addition to Windows and is capable of handling much larger spreadsheets than many other programs, making it a good choice for people working with large amounts of data.

K-Spread (Kuma Computers)

Part of the GEM based series of products from Kuma Computers, K-Spread offers a reasonable number of functions for its price.

DATABASES

There are two main types of databases – relational and flat file. A relational database makes it a lot easier to cross-reference information. If you are working with lots of information or accessing data on the college mainframe, support for SQL (Structured Query Language) may be useful. Screen and report painting allow you to draw forms on the screen rather than having to program them manually. For sensitive applications, consider a package that allows you to assign passwords to data. Although network versions of most packages are available, some come with support built in. The maximum amount of data that you can hold is decided by the limits in the tables, but unless you have a very large application, you will not need to worry too much about them.

DOS applications

Cardbox (Business Simulations)

Cardbox allows the creation of freeform databases based on card files. Any word, number or date on the card can be indexed and the cards can be formatted into different fields, with up to 36 lines and 132 columns.

DataEase (DataEase Ltd)

DataEase provides an easy to use menu system as well as a powerful command language. Complex applications can be created without having to do any programming.

DataPerfect (WordPerfect UK)

New features include a printing feature which queues and spools reports, improved documentation and improved network performance. Compatible with other WordPerfect products but the inability to read dBase files may be a serious drawback for some users.

dBase (Borland)

dBase 6 is based on the dBase language which is an industry standard. New features include easier database design, Query By Example and an application generator.

Delta 5 (Compsoft Plc)

Delta 5 is a flexible package allowing straightforward construction of databases to handle transactions and similar tasks. An unlimited number of record hierarchies can be related, each up to 18 billion records.

Demon (Transaction Point)

Demon is a powerful database in its own right but it can be used alongside ICL's integral office system and can run on Unix or mainframe computers.

FoxBase+ (Fox Software International)

Foxbase+ is a flexible package based on the dBase language including an application generator, soundex searching and automatic documentation generation.

FoxPro (Fox Software International)

FoxPro is both fast and flexible. It is compatible with dBase but has more functions and is a popular choice for developing database applications.

Magic II (Magic Software Enterprises)

MSE prefers to describe this package as an applications generator which can be linked directly to mainframes if necessary, rather than as a simple relational database.

Oracle Database 6 (Oracle Corporation UK)

Often used to develop applications in other platforms such as Unix, VMS, HP MPE/XL and so on. Package includes SQL forms, SQL menu,

SQL report writer, proSQL and a number of utilities including a database administration tool.

Paradox (Borland)

Paradox is a powerful package including automatic network support and a WYSIWYG reports generator. The built-in application language can be enhanced through the use of an SQL option.

PC-File (OpenSoft)

PC-File is a low cost, flexible package that provides built-in charting functions and letter writing for easy production of merged mail shots. Soundex searching allows easy retrieval of data based on phonetic information.

Personal RBase (Microrim)

This package allows easy creation of applications and queries through the use of pull-down menus and supports a mouse, allowing you to point and click at options and data.

Progress 4GL/RDBMS (Progress Software)

Also available as a Windows version, Progress is a database development package with a language (4GL), a relational database management system and a library of end-user tools.

RBase 3.1 (Microrim)

RBase supplies the same mouse support and pull-down menus as the personal version of the product, together with fully integrated SQL and the ability to record oft-performed operations as scripts.

SmartWare II (Informix Software)

The SmartWare database manager is part of the SmartWare integrated package and is supplied with the Smart communications module and programming language to allow the construction of complex applications.

SuperDB (Computer Associates)

SuperDB provides a programmable macro facility for the creation of applications and the ability to create graphs from databases. An unlimited number of simultaneous search criteria can be applied.

Windows and graphical applications

dBFast (Computer Associates)

dBFast is a compiler, not a database. It turns dBase source code into applications that run under Windows. It is strictly a developer's tool not intended for the casual, interactive database user.

Formbase (Ventura Software)

Formbase allows easy construction of Windows-based databases using forms drawn on the screen. Graphics images from other Windows applications can be included in your database. A selection of form templates is included.

Omnis 7 (Blyth Software)

Omnis 5 has been completely rewritten for this version, but all applications developed in the old version will be converted to 7. The package's workings might seem idiosyncratic, but Omnis fans praise its power.

SuperBase 4 Windows (Precision Software)

SuperBase allows the inclusion of graphical images in a database and provides a command language that allows you to program menu-base applications. LAN and communication features allow easy sharing of data between users.

Window Base (Software Products International)

Window Base is fully WYSIWYG and supports Windows DDE for exchange of data with other applications. Images can be included in the databases. SQL queries can be constructed through dialogue boxes and push buttons or by direct entry.

K-Data (Kuma Computers)

K-Data is one of the K series of Kuma products, including K-Spread, K-Graph and K-Word, all running under GEM. Data can be exchanged easily between them.

DESKTOP PUBLISHING

The programs listed here range from simple packages that allow you to produce a party invitation to complex ones capable of producing a magazine. If you want a professional quality output, you need a package that will produce colour separations. Support for the Pantone colour matching system means that printed colours will match those shown on the screen. Many professional typesetters use PostScript, which will give you access to a wide range of typefaces. Kerning and tracking control – the spacing of lines and letters on the page – and hyphenation control will let you specify where words should be split. If you are working on long documents it may save time to opt for features like a spellchecker and search and replace. Some systems will even create an index or table of contents for you.

DOS applications

Jetsetter (Garbo Systems)

Originally designed specifically for producing high-quality output on a Laser-Jet compatible printer, this program now supports many other printer standards.

PageMaker (Aldus)

One of the most powerful DTP packages on the market, PageMaker is the standard by which many others are judged. Files are compatible with DOS and Macintosh versions of the program.

Publisher (Microsoft)

This is a cheap but powerful package that comes with a set of Page Wizards to help you create documents easily. A wide range of graphics formats can be imported.

Ventura Publisher (Ventura Software)

This is the Windows version of a package that was originally written for the GEM operating system. It provides almost all the features necessary for professional DTP work, though it lacks Pantone colour.

Windows and graphical applications

Deskpress (GST Software)

One of the more flexible of the GEM based DTP packages. Deskpress is supplied with Typografica fonts and a selection of predefined style sheets.

Finesse (Logi UK)

GEM and a black and white image library are included in the cost of the package. Finesse will handle documents up to 99 pages long.

GEM Desktop Publisher (Digital Research)

In spite of its price, this package lacks some of the functions necessary for the serious user, such as the ability to produce colour separations.

Timeworks Publisher (GST Software Products)

Timeworks is a versatile product that is supplied with the Typografica Prime collection of typefaces and support for downloadable fonts on both PostScript and laser jet printers.

GRAPHICS PACKAGES

These packages fall into two main categories – presentation graphics and drawing packages. Presentation packages are designed for creating slides or screens while drawing packages are more general purpose. If you want slides or drawings completed professionally, you should look for a package that supports PostScript and colour separations. The number of colours available varies with your type of display or your Windows set-up.

DOS applications

DrawPerfect (WordPerfect UK)

DrawPerfect is a full-feature presentation package that allows the creation of images from PlanPerfect spreadsheets and other information sources.

Foxgraph (Fox Software International)

This package can create a wide range of graphs from a selection of database packages. Graphs can be exported to most major DTP packages.

Freelance Graphics (Lotus Developments UK)

Freelance for DOS provides many features and has an interface reminiscent of the Lotus 1-2-3 spreadsheet. Compared to some other programs, the range of file formats is a little limited.

Harvard Graphics (Software Publishing Corporation)

Harvard Graphics is the leading presentation graphics package for DOS. It has charting facilities, the ability to produce pie charts, graphs and a range of other technical diagrams. It also has extensive presentation capabilities.

Windows and graphical applications

Arts and Letters (Roderick Manhatten)

This package provides a wide selection of drawing tools, including the ability to turn text into curves for editing. Charting and bitmap trace facilities are provided.

Charisma (Micrografx)

This package features good file import and export capabilities and can be used with its slide show manager for simple presentations.

Corel Draw! (Frontline Distribution)

A flexible drawing package, this program provides a wide range of tools for manipulating both text and images.

Cricket Graph (Computer Associates)

Cricket Graph was designed to allow the easy conversion of data into graphics, with a selection of 12 predefined graph formats and WYSIWYG display.

Cricket Presents (Computer Associates)

Cricket Presents provides the ability to create free-standing slide shows. Spreadsheet files can be imported but not databases.

Designworks (Electric Distribution)

Designworks creates drawings, diagrams, logos and charts. It comes with a library of clip art images and you can save your own drawings to a customized library.

Freelance Graphics for Windows (Lotus Developments UK)

Freelance for Windows provides a 'SmartMasters' design environment which allows you to just fill in the blanks of your presentation. The package is supplied with a large library of clip art images.

Harvard Draw (Software Publishing Corporation)

Creates illustrations for reports, newsletters, flyers or presentations. Twelve preset palettes, each containing 150 colours per palette, plus user defined palettes are supported. Full WYSIWYG text entry.

Harvard Graphics for Windows (Software Publishing Corporation)

The Windows version of the Harvard Graphics package includes video compression technology, allowing live multimedia images to be incorporated into presentations.

Hollywood (IBM UK)

This is a powerful and fairly easy to use presentation graphics package but slightly limited in the number of fonts that are supported.

PowerPoint (Micrografx)

PowerPoint provides a range of over 16 million colours and an extensive selection of graphics tools, together with wordprocessing features and the ability to generate hand-outs to accompany your slide presentations.

Windows Draw (Micrografx)

Draw provides a wide range of tools, support for 24 bit colour and an extensive library of clip art, including political figures and geographical information.

Other applications

Artline (Digital Research)

An illustration tool with which you can manipulate text for headlines and logos or create illustrations for presentations.

Davrelle (GST Software Products)

Davrelle allows the easy creation of graphs and slide shows from both spreadsheets and database files. The package provides the ability to update graphs automatically when the original data is changed.

Appendix 3
Shareware

This appendix offers brief descriptions of some of the shareware programs that are available and that will be of use to a variety of health care professionals. Remember that shareware is not free. The concept of shareware allows you to try programs before you pay a fee to the author which covers your regular use of the program. The fee often brings you a new version of the program and a telephone support system. The concept of shareware depends on users making such payments to the authors of the programs. Note, however, that you are free to distribute copies of shareware programs to other people. They, in turn, must pay a fee to the author if they continue to use the program. There are sometimes special registration rates for institutions and educational establishments. Health care professionals who like the idea of shareware and want to use a range of it should investigate this aspect.

ORGANIZATIONAL PROGRAMS

There are a number of commercial organizer programs on the market that take over the work of diaries and of project management. There are also some excellent shareware programs that do the job just as well.

Tie Database

A Time/Income/Expense system for a self-employed professional or small business. Assists in filling out taxes, evalutes profit/loss situations, provides audit trail and accurate time utilization. Uses pop-up screens. dBase 3 and 3+ compatible.

In Control

Tracks appointments, commitments, callbacks, has freeform data search, roladex features, label management, and reports. Handles label creation for multiple countries, has intelligent phone dialling system, built-in proposal/invoice generator.

PC-Label Maker

Simple program allows you to create labels, then print them in different fonts, in 1, 2, or 3 columns, and any number of times. Has online help screens and is very easy to use.

Client & Note File

Excellent dedicated program. Allows you to add, edit, delete and view notes and clients. Search and generate reports by fields. Quick and easy to use interface and data entry screen.

Statistics/Data Analysis

STATA is a program for manipulating, displaying and analysing data. Easy to use and extremely powerful. Can be operated from the command line or has a complete menu driven interface.

Personal Appointment Locat

Allows you to organize appointments, provides online help, shows secular and religious holidays automatically, allows you to customize the program to your needs and style, will produce a calendar for any month, and much more.

Decision Analysis System

Designed for individuals faced with the problem of choosing between comparable items. Enter facts, stats, preferences, features, prices, etc. along with weight value (what each aspect is worth) into custom database, program rates, gives recommendations.

Personal Calendar

Displays a 3 month scrollable calendar, a running analogue and digital clock and a time oriented event list/note list. Warnings and alarms notify when something is pending or overdue. Notes and tracking info can be printed.

Ample Notice

Calendar/alarm program. Enter coming or cycling (monthly, yearly, etc.) events to have the computer remind you. Pop-up reminders no matter what computer is running. Prints notes in various formats including compressed for wallet size.

Managing People

Self-help tool for managers. Combines tutorials and tests on managing concerns. Covers communications, delegation, boss/employee evaluation, positive attitudes, decision making, motivating employees, planning improvement, interviews, getting things done.

Pop Form

Programmable TSR program allows you to grab info from the screen, then print it on a pre-made form. You can actually print your forms with any info you can find on the screen from within any program.

Business Cards

This simple program will allow you to easily make your own business cards. Automatically justifies text left, right or centre. Uses different fonts and borders.

Active Life

Outstanding commercial quality software. Powerful system for planning, managing and tracking one's active business and personal life. Dynamic schedules manage workflow effectively, recurring activities need be entered only once.

Easy Project

Tool to assist anyone who manages. Facilitates planning, scheduling and tracking of all types of projects. Up to 2000 tasks per project, Gantt charts, auto scheduling, extensive reporting, context-sensitive help, and much more.

The Day Care Manager

An incredibly detailed day care management package. It covers nearly every conceivable need for a day care program of any size. Complete client/child information database, payment tracking, complete accounting.

The Volunteer Network

Designed to computerize volunteers' skills, experiences and assignments. It tracks volunteer information, year-to-date and total award hours, dollar value of hours worked, and scheduled assignments.

The Donor Network

For tracking donations in a variety of ways. Handles cash donations, pledges and user-definable periodic billing. It stores donor information including contact names and secondary addresses.

Med Number 1

A new medical office management system for increasing efficiency in the daily administration of medical practices. No special forms are needed for printing; all reports print on 8½" by 11" paper.

Dental Number 1

Handles statements, patient ledgers, superbill and insurance forms, daily charges, receipts, month-to-date summary, ageing accounts, and more.

Sitter

Full-featured placement service for baby sitters and respite care. Features weekly scheduling, unlimited job orders per patron, match job to sitter, full accounts receivable, general ledger, statements, and more.

CALCULATORS

Every computer user needs a calculator program. Although the right hand side of the keyboard looks as though it offers computing functions, software is required to make it work in this way. These are just a couple of the many calculator programs that are available as shareware.

The Statistician

Statistics calculator. Regression analysis, data transformations, descriptive statistics, time series forecasting, random samples, data sort and more.

Scientific Calculator

Program to perform scientific calculations. Does unit conversions, mensuration, complex, physical formulas, trig, matrix, and general functions, function evaluations and statistics.

COMPUTER HELP PROGRAMS

As we noted in Chapters 2 and 4, it is necessary to get to grips with DOS if you are going to work with personal computers in any depth. These programs are an excellent way of learning about the operating system.

Help-DOS

Provides a quick reference for DOS commands and programs. Allows user to add his own text files to be accessed by Help-DOS. Has two versions, command line and memory resident. To use, simply enter HELP DOSCOMMAND, Help will display the proper syntax.

Computer Glossary

A 73k file containing a glossary of common and not so common computer terms. Listed alphabetically, very comprehensive.

Tutor Com

Interactive DOS tutorial. Teaches, asks questions, prompts for answers. Covers nine subjects: keyboards, computer history, introduction to computers/binary numbers and the CPU, I/O devices, DOS, subdirectories, batch files, structured programming.

Computer Tutor

Highly recommended for new computer users. Text file covering some of the useful, little known aspects of DOS. Covers the CONFIG.SYS file, AUTOEXEC.BAT, PATHS, COMMAND.COM, ANSI, batch files, PROMPT=, the environment and more.

Hyper-DOS

Hypertext DOS command manual. Quickly locate related DOS commands. Very comprehensive, supplies syntax info, usage and descriptions for all DOS commands. Find information by following commands to related commands. Bookmark feature, educational, with many features.

DOS Summary

Starting the program will display an alphabetical listing of DOS commands. Choose one for full description and command syntax. Start the program followed with a DOS command and it will display information for that command.

Batch File Tutorial

Everything you have ever wanted to know about batch files but were afraid to ask. Shows you how to create or modify batch files. Also includes an editor to create your batch files.

Disk Consultant

A software package that includes valuable information about computer cleaning and maintenance, speeding up your machine, hardware and software buyer's guide, 800 and fax number directories.

FREEFORM DATABASE PROGRAMS

As we noted in Chapter 6, freeform databases are ideal for handling unstructured data of various sorts. Also, as we saw in the last chapter of the book, freeform databases can be used to analyse qualitative data in research projects.

Index Card Filer

Index card type database with many features. Enter name and address, phone number and comments. Search, merge, print, sort and more. Nice interface.

Get It

Freeform database and reminder program. Well written program with many options; find word/phrase or related words/phrases, remind, edit, view, add, import, export, many print options, shell to DOS, context-sensitive help, various utilities.

Mini Db

A program to create and manage a database. Very fast and friendly, includes an extensive template library and good documentation.

Easy-Base

Extremely easy to use database. Easy interface allows you to design forms and reports, do string searches, create sorted files. Offers on-line help, data compression and much more.

Freebase

A freeform database featuring data entry from any ASCII text editor, rapid search, print search results or write to disk, keywords to link records, shell to DOS, reports, good documentation. Maximum 100 records with data file of approximately 45k.

Freefile

This is a flat database program. Up to 2 billion records; up to ten indexes per database; records can be 1000 characters long; each record can have 100 fields; fields can be up to 65 characters, etc.

Fastfile 2

A small, fast, simple database program that's just right for beginners and small businesses with laptops or single floppy disk computers. It also works on a hard drive.

Information Please

Freeform database program allows you to store various length records (i.e. paragraphs) and search, display and print them according to keyword matches.

FULL DATABASE SYSTEMS

Full database programs are usually very expensive. Here are some excellent shareware programs that are often as good as their commercial counterparts.

File Express

File Express is an information management program. It allows easy manipulation of small and medium sized databases using menu-driven commands. Allows you to create and maintain files of almost any type.

Zephyr

Fully relational, FoxPro compatible database management system for non-programmers. Up to 25 databases can be manipulated simultaneously. Its performance is roughly 16 times that of dBase III and eight times that of dBase IV. Applications (including reports, labels, lists and form letters) can be designed and generated in minutes, not months. Quick and easy database applications.

PC-File

ButtonWare's upgraded PC-File 5.01 supports dBase III plus file format, LANs and five types of graphs generated by the program using data you specify. Has context-sensitive help, interactive teach mode, maximum of 1 billion records with 70 fields each.

Profile

This is a new, powerful database program with special functions for mailing lists. Sort, search and bulk mail sort. Produce reports, labels, mailmerge files. Functions include unlimited database files, flexible form set-up, relational look-up capabilities, telephone dialler, 150 fields per record, 3000 characters per record, up to ten index fields per database, and more.

DESKTOP PUBLISHING PROGRAMS

Commercial desktop publishing programs are amongst the most powerful and expensive of all computer programs. Here are some shareware offerings.

City Desk

Simple desktop publishing. You write the text file, then let City Desk print it. Prints in 1, 2 or 3 columns, shell to DOS, justify text, incorporate graphics, 11 print styles, auto index creation and much more. Excellent printing enhancement program.

Rubicon Publisher

Comprehensive publisher modelled on typesetting concepts with over 120 features. Supports 200+ printers including 9/24 pin dot matrix, LaserJet and PostScript. Comes with two font families, supports scalable LJ-III and PS fonts, has VGA (mono or colour), preview to display files before printing. Comes with a step-by-step tutorial and a concise manual that documents all features. Supports GEM.IMG bitmap graphics. Operates on plain ASCII files by imbedding tags in the document.

Code to Code

A collection of programs designed to move, delete or translate codes from various DTP, wordprocessors and typesetter files. Allows a user to edit files without the codes then re-insert the codes, creating a new document.

SPECIALIST HEALTH CARE PROGRAMS

Many of these programs are American in origin and this may have to be borne in mind when considering these programs for use in the UK.

Drug Interaction Program

Enter a drug name then the program will display the drugs that interact with it. It also gives a description of the effects the combination will have on the human body. Has about 60 000 listings. Works well but has a simple text interface.

Prescription Assistant

Designed to assist the physician in daily practice by producing printed prescriptions. Improves speed, legibility, documentation, versatility and alteration security. Handles from one to 100 physicians. Nice interface.

Health Risk Appraisal

Professional software from the Center for Disease Control. Asks a series of lifestyle, location, attitude and medical questions to create a printed report estimating your chances of survival in a ten year period. Very comprehensive, reports look professional.

Flower Remedy Finder

Database of flower remedies. Based on the work of English physician Edward Bach, who compiled a list of 38 flowers whose essences were found to effect cures for emotional and physiological problems. Select problems from large list to find cures.

Non-Medical Pain Relief

Learn how to help yourself and your clients relieve pain with accupressure, massage and other techniques. Pictures and text tutorial.

Appendix 3

SPREADSHEET PROGRAMS

Again, many of these shareware spreadsheet programs can do most of the functions that are offered in commercial packages.

PC-Calc Plus

Buttonware's powerful improved spreadsheet. Has graphics, split screens, 8087/80287 support, DOS access, macros, DOS path support, supports Hercules, CGA, EGA, VGA, sophisticated time/date functions, 20 maths functions, six logical functions (if then/true/false, etc.), 14 special functions (bessel function, hyperbolic cosine/sine/tangent, etc.), six statistical functions, 15 trigonometric functions, 200 page manual on disk.

Turbo Calc

An integrated spreadsheet, and pull-down menu, file editor. Spreadsheet size 8192 rows × 2 columns to 90 rows × 256 columns. Has many maths and financial functions and graphics capability. Editor features word-wrap, search, block, and more.

EZ-Spreadsheet

Another in the series of EZ programs. (All EZ programs use the same pull-down window interface.) 64 columns × 512 rows, compatible with most other spreadsheets, add, subtract, multiply, divide, do what-if routines, online help, and much more. Easy to learn and use.

Express Calc

Express Calc is an easy-to-use 'visible spreadsheet' program. If you work with numbers, at home or at work, this is a very straightforward and useful spreadsheet program.

Proqube Lite

This 5-star spreadsheet has all the functions of Lotus 1-2-3 but in 3D format. Lets you view your data in six different ways. Import and export Lotus, dBase and more. Graphs, macros, etc.

Quickplan

A memory resident spreadsheet program. Handy for popping up when you are in another program.

VIRUS PROTECTION PROGRAMS

As we noted in Chapter 4, protection against computer viruses is essential. Here are some shareware virus protection programs.

SS Choice

Can be configured to protect all classes of files (COM, EXE, BAT, TXT, etc.) and boot sector. Provides CRC (checksum) protection algorithm and TSR program protection. Identifies attacking programs by name.

MS-DOS Anti Virus

MS-DOS anti virus protection. Uses CRC to check IO.SYS, MS DOS.SYS, COMMAND.COM, CONFIG.SYS and AUTOEXEC.BAT.

Virus Detector

Uses two separate CRC algorithms for comparison. Creates three files containing info for up to five directories (Old, New and Report). Can read every byte of info to seek out a virus.

Vaccine and Virus Detector

Virus protection. Detects viruses, then removes them automatically. Then rechecks for possible damage elsewhere and corrects that too.

Anti-Virus Programs

Collection of more than 15 virus protection programs. Some search for and remove viruses, others prevent deletes and formats, others do other things. Includes BOMBSQAD, CHK4BOMB, FLU-SHOT, HDSENTRY, TRAPDISK, VACINE, TROJAN, NOVIRUS, and others.

File-Check

Preventive program provides sure protection against viruses. Makes a snapshot of all your files' attributes and FAT info (date, time, size, etc.). Alerts you to changes that occur when you run them again. Requires more time to use than some other programs but is claimed to be virtually foolproof.

WINDOWS SHAREWARE PROGRAMS

There are some high quality shareware programs available for use with Windows and the selection is increasing all the time.

Screen Peace

Excellent, multi-featured screen saver for Windows v3.0. Over 15 animated screens selected randomly when you cease using the keyboard. Aquarium, puzzle, outer space, moving clock and many more.

Easel

A Microsoft Windows program for displaying, manipulating and converting various picture formats.

Command Post and Browser

CP easily personalizes executive control window. Add dropdown menu items, execute application items from the menus, screen blanking, copy, move, delete and more. Requires Windows v2.03 or newer. Browser displays text, prints, copies to clipboard.

Windows Clock

Displays time and date in multiple formats, has two alarms, 'remembers' its screen position, has two stopwatches and two countdown timers, context-sensitive help and is screen saver compatible.

Wsmooth

Smooth scrolling file viewer for Windows 3.0. Allows you to control the speed of scrolling. The smooth scroll makes it easy to read even while it's moving. Simple and useful.

Windows Post-It

Electronic Post-It Notes. Allows you to 'stick' various sizes of yellow notes on your Windows screen. The notes' position and contents are remembered when Windows is exited so they are still there when you return.

Paint Shop

Complete Windows graphics file viewer, converter and screen capture utility. PS will display, convert, alter and print TIFF, GIF, WPG, BMP,

PCX, MAC, IMG and RLE graphics. Altering includes stretch/shrink, trim, rotate, flip, dithering and more.

Aporia

A fully graphical, object-oriented user interface which lets you customize your working environment. It's a better way to organize your work by allowing you to display graphically your programs and data files.

WinEdit

An ASCII text editor designed to take full advantage of the Windows 3.0 graphical environment. WinEdit is first and foremost a programmer's editor, with features designed for creating and maintaining program source code.

Winbatch

Windows 3.0 batch language. Allows you to create sophisticated batch language files to control your Windows environment. It has over 100 different functions to manipulate files, directories, windows, and other Windows applications.

WORDPROCESSING PROGRAMS

As with database and spreadsheet programs, the best of the shareware wordprocessing programs match a number of commercial packages.

Mind Reader

Full-featured wordprocessor with A1 capabilities. Learns your style. Autosave, dictionary, special dictionary for often used words and phrases, Instaspell, line drawing, calculator, easy to use, much more. Great for 'hunt and peck' typists.

Galaxy

Fast RAM-based wordprocessor. Offers most standard wordprocessing features while being easy to use and learn. Keyboard commands and pull-down menus, macro record, dictionary, Windows additional files, shell to DOS, and much more.

Scribe

Unique wordprocessor offering basic wordprocessing features and the ability to analyse and advise on your style of writing. Gives effective writing suggestions for various age levels and a graphic view of your style.

PC-Write

Quicksoft's outstanding wordprocessor. Has all the usual plus some interesting extras like shorthand mode (create files using abbreviated words, the program reassembles using your list), DOS commands, supports over 500 printers, easy font insertion, display various text colours on screen, many box drawing options, auto line numbering, various file filters, footnotes, easy index/contents creation, print while editing, record key strokes, shell to DOS, window multiple files, typewriter mode, 50 000 word spellchecker, WordStar compatible, cut and paste, parallel column format editing, network support, online help (45 screens). Tutorial and help guide. One of the best wordprocessors on the market, either shareware or commercial.

Chiwrit

Multifont wordprocessor giving true WYSIWYG. Has up to ten fonts and 250 super/subscript levels per line. Has popular printer support and prints in both HI/LO resolution. Has most of the standard features. Unique wordprocessor.

EZ-Write

RAM-based wordprocessor offers the best features while being easy to use and learn. Has pull-down menus with CNTRL key counterparts. Has find and replace, online help, paragraph formatting, justified text, easy print code entry, block commands and much more.

PC-Type 4

Virtual rewrite of the excellent PC-Type II. Many new and enhanced features, extensive mail merge features, 100 000 word dictionary, catches misspelled words and offers replacements, view up to ten different files simultaneously, context-sensitive help, pull-down menus or commands, supports calculations, box drawing features, macros, move and copy within/between files. Has search and replace, align and sort columns,

DOS command support, WHOOPS key, headers/footers, date and time stamps, file bookmarks, full featured label processing, multiple default settings, save all or parts of files, visually line up columns, compatibility with PC-Calc+, PC-File 5.0, extensive graphing features. Much more yet easy to use and learn.

New York Word

Easy to use, full-featured wordprocessor. Features pull-down menus, spellchecker, macros, footnoting, mail merge, index and table of contents generation, cut and paste, box drawing, calculator, good printer support and much more.

H-Key

H-Key is a writing tool for the severely motor impaired who wish to write. H-Key uses a single key entry principle for entering text. Comes with complete documentation.

PC-Outline

Allows you to deal with ideas like you would deal with words. You can organize, categorize, arrange, rearrange and manipulate your ideas. This is one that everyone should try.

GRAPHICS PROGRAMS

These are some of the graphics programs that are available. Some of them are not so fully featured as the commercially available ones but many offer excellent value.

Optiks

Optiks is a 'jack of all trades' graphics program. Can read/write/alter more than 25 different formats (.art, .bas, .bsg, .cut, .iff, .gif, .img, .pic, and more). Merge, print, image (change size/shape), draw, dither, scan, five fonts and much more.

Pronto Graph

Graphing made easy and flexible. Combines graphing features with rudimentary paint program. Uses three 'layers' to store images (graph/

paint/text). Features online help, grids, lines, points, bar menus, and spike graphs, 21 background patterns.

Leonardo

Full-featured graphics editor. Creates 4-colour graphics/icon screens and files. Features online help, slide show, size, style, circle, boxes, shadow, zoom, mottle, outline, paint, reverse, exchange colours and more. Files are easily added to basic programs.

Icon-Maker

Dot graphics program for making icons. Supports 640X200, 320X200 and 160X100 graphics modes. Data can be put directly into the program data area.

PC Picture Graphics

Excellent program for creating/printing graphic screens. Has hundreds of pictures (zodiac, music, signs, maths, equipment, vehicles, flowchart, misc, animals, more), a variety of fonts, many drawing tools. Supports joystick and popular printers. Easy to use.

Screen Designer

Tool for designing screen displays. Has line draw, auto-box, and a special programmer's interface, can export displays into most languages. Supports HERC, CGA, EGA, PGA, and mono. Compatible with IBM graphic printers and compatibles.

Hi-Res Rainbow

Full-featured CGA paint package. Pull-down windows, icons, supports joystick/mouse/keyboard/tablet, ray, zoom, spray, brush, box, fill, circle, arc, symmetry mode, reflexing, move, smear, rainbow (scrolls colours in background) and much, much more.

Slide Generator

Produce medium quality slides or transparencies for use with overhead projector. Images can be saved, edited, created, displayed or printed. The output is put on paper and you can then photograph for slides or copy onto transparency material.

Edraw

Drawing program for technical people like engineers, teachers and students. Besides drawing lines, boxes, circles and symbols, includes logic/electronic symbols. Draw schematics, block diagrams, flowcharts and features automatic panning.

Colour Paint Graphics Package

Complete paint program for medium and high-resolution graphics PCs. The system comes with good documentation and will support graphics printers like Epson. Many help screens.

Symbol Design

Symbol Design is a personal computer designing package, with a spreadsheet type menu that makes it easy to bring up, create and mix symbols, fonts, and shapes for professional looking presentations.

THERAPEUTIC AND HEALTH RELATED PROGRAMS

These are some programs that relate specifically to the health care field.

Sign Friends and Learn to Sign

Two programs which use animated graphics to display and teach signing, the sign language used by many deaf people. Covers phrases, letters and words. Sign Friends requires BASIC.

Big-WP

A memory-resident context-sensitive display enlarger specially designed for use with WordPerfect and LetterPerfect. Works with versions 5.0, 5.1 and LP 1.0. Enlarges text within WP (only screen portions with text).

B-Edit

Multi-featured, large character text editor, 60 000 word spellchecker, multiple size screen fonts, block functions, window 2 files, search and replace, word-wrap, online help and more.

B-Pop

Memory-resident magnifying glass. Pops up over the text mode screens of other software and enlarges them, making them easier to read. Has three different screen fonts and online help. Use arrow keys to move around enlarged text.

B-Ware

A collection of four big text utilities. B-Dir displays directory sorted or portioned, B-Type works like DOS's TYPE command, B-Look scrolls text files, B-Print prints ASCII text files in large type fonts.

Baby Watch

Allows you to calculate or enter the date of conception then records the date and gives you a graphic (text) description of the baby's formation in the womb. Very interesting for families-to-be. Provides descriptions for each stage of pregnancy.

COMPUTER UTILITY PROGRAMS

Everyone uses these sorts of programs at some time. They are often tiny programs that do something very specific, such as help you to transfer files from one disk to another. There is a huge range of utility programs available and these are just some of that selection.

Arcmaster

Support program for five popular archiving utilities. Creates a visual shell to make the features of each program easier to use. Supports ARC, ARCA/ARCE, PKPAK/PKUNPAK, PAK and PKZIP/PKUNZIP. ASP.

PK Ware

Using the ZIP format this program allows you to compress files into one archived file. Sometimes compresses more than 50%, offers fast compression, self-extracting files, and a variety of compression methods.

An Ounce of Prevention

A generational file protection and recovery system that automatically maintains up to eight generations of all your critical files. In addition it protects your hard disk drive from accidental or malicious formats.

Flexibak Plus

A flexible, easy to use hard disk back-up system that takes a logical, simple and unique approach to the back-up problem. You only need to take a full back-up once and then all subsequent back-ups are placed on the same back-up disks.

DirBack

DirBack creates directories and copies the files to and from any drive. The result of backing up your entire hard drive is a set of floppies that duplicates all of the directories and files the way they exist on your hard disk.

Offload

Designed to perform data archiving and retrieval for PCs in a manner similar to the mainframe world. Allows the user to archive files from the hard drive to floppies for permanent storage.

Stowaway

Stowaway moves inactive files to offline disk storage, giving you room on your hard disk while still maintaining instant access to all your data. Lots of features with a very user-friendly menu.

PC-MAG Benchmark

The PC-MAG benchmark test set. Allows you to thoroughly test computer systems using a set of 17 diagnostic programs. Test memory, video, I/O, drives, just about everything. All programs operate from a central menu. Use this before you buy a new system.

Disk Efficiency

Measures the storage efficiency of any group of files on any floppy/hard disk supported by MS-DOS.

Set-Up and System Utilities

Several programs for testing system speeds and hard drive set-up. Clock 'real world' system speeds, perform hard disk drive partition selection and format.

Test Drive

Professional software to analyse your floppy drives' performance. Provides continuous test for real time adjustments, tells you when to clean drives, test alignment, spindle speed, read/write, hysteresis, head azimuth, hub centring, more.

Total System Statistics

Run to display total system stats. Reports date, time, DOS version, system type, processor type, co-processor type, memory size, expanded memory size, free memory, ROM BIOS, number of/type of ports, much more.

Hard Disk Diagnostics

Extensive HD diagnostics program. Two types of test, destructive and non-destructive. Provides complete information on how your hard drive is performing and can complete high level format.

Visual System Information

Run VSI to display a graphic image of any computer's system configuration.

HDTest 5.35 and DirEdit

Thoroughly tests your hard drive for errors and impending errors, marks any found as bad and moves data occupying bad sectors to good sectors. DirEdit rearranges directories and/or files.

System Speed Test

Real time system test graphically displays CPU speed, video speed, maths speed (trig functions, simple identifiers, array elements, array passing, conditional jumps, video timing, and five more maths functions). Use to compare various computer systems.

DOS SHELLS

As we noted in Chapter 2, DOS shells can simplify the management of your computer. At their simplest, they offer a simple menu system that pops up on the screen every time you start the computer. More elaborate shells have file copying, deleting and transfer facilities. Some have calculators and notebooks built in.

Automenu

Program allows you to create custom menus for your programs. Many features, password protection, chained menus, unattended execution, supports all video, mouse support, can be configured memory resident, auto menu make feature and more.

Power Menu

Super hard disk manager. Password protection, submenus, screen saver, pop-up DOS window, dBase II comp., search, copy, move, delete, set clock, define colours. Will read hard drive and automatically create menus.

Directory Maintenance

Yet another DOS shell program. Has all the usual features, copy, delete, make/delete directories, move, run, view, search, sort and more. The difference in this program is it's easy to use, intuitive interface. Good looking and well thought out program.

Hard Disk Menu

A DOS shell that hides the operating system, yet does not get in the way of the experienced user. Up to 100 menu files with ten pages each, online help, mouse support, macros, phone set-up, run files, user configurable titles and much more.

Still River Shell

Powerful DOS enhancement for file and directory management. Eliminate most file name and command typing, display graphic tree, find files, find text within files, copy/move/delete, view files, sort, back up to floppies, buffer DOS commands and much more.

Stupendos

Outstanding DOS shell. Copy, view, move, delete, unzip, sort, execute, change attributes and display GIFs. Has online help, pull-down menus, disk stats, allows tagging of files, directory tree, mouse support, finds text and is very easy to use.

Easy Access

Create stand-alone menu systems. Configure colours, headings, titles, etc. Many features, screen blanker, calendar, clock, reminder subsystem (reminds you of coming/current events), password security, user sign on, no memory overhead and more.

Jobs

Job Organization and Back-up System. Hard disk manager, DOS shell, utility set, menu manager and more. Multi-featured program allows you to run programs, copy, delete, rename, etc., print, search, sort, compare data, and automate frequently performed operations.

Tree Top

Fast and easy file manager. Many features, execute files, pull-down menus, sort files, copy, move, rename, delete and print files, mouse support, tag by date/attributes, file/text search, complete manual, prompt for full disks, run editor and much more.

Windos

A graphical 'Windows-like' menu program for DOS. Customizable program icons (colours, size), mouse support, customizable clocks (size, colours, digital, analogue, etc.), built-in screen blanker and more. Good looking menu.

Scout-Em

A memory-resident disk/directory/file manager and DOS shell that can be invoked from the DOS level or from within an active program. Has over 30 functions. Uses 65k of RAM. Runs from expanded memory.

Dosamatic Task-Switching

Task-switching utility that allows the user several programs for the purpose of manipulating them with simple keystroke commands. It contains a nice menu that lists available drives, directories and files on the current drive.

File Commando

File management. Provides a menu-driven environment for showing directory tree, sorts files, creates subdirectories, formats disks, changes attributes, print spooler, and more.

PC Desk Team

PC Desk Team features calendars, full function calculator, alarm clock, time displays, hourly chime, notepad, phone book, typewriter emulator, printer controls. Memory resident. DOS command access.

Treeview

A hard disk and file maintenance utility system. Can be used with automenu or as a stand-alone program. You can also run this from floppy disk drives. It removes the guesswork from file maintenance.

PA Menu Manager

Some of the features included are DOS functions like disk formatting, copy files, etc., notepad, memory status, calculator, wordprocessor, phone directory, phone/modem set-up, video select, extended memory usage.

Menu Master

Small enough to be used on disks but is mainly intended for a hard drive. Easy to use with up to 24 menu selections plus things like password protection, personalize the menu title, customize colours, and more.

Graphical Menu System

A graphical menu system that allows you to use your computer more quickly, easily and more intuitively. Complex DOS commands are replaced by easy-to-use command buttons, pop-up windows and dialogue boxes. Lots of features.

EZ Menu

Offers full mouse support to access menu items as well as utilities and functions. Menus may contain up to 18 individual items with unlimited submenus. Contains a datebook function that can be used as a diary or reminder system.

Dosmenu

A DOS menuing program. It allows you to set up a list of options on a menu, and commands for each of those options. Handy for the knowledgeable user who is setting up a system for a less knowledgeable user.

Bibliography

Adamson, M. (1990) *Small Real-Time Systems Design*, Sigma Press, Wilmslow.

Allen, J. (1989) *How to Develop Your Personal Management Skills*, Kogan Page, London.

Ashworth, P. (1987) Technology and machines – bad masters but good servants. *Intensive Care Nursing*, **3**(1), 1–2.

Ball, M.J. and Hannah, K.J. (1984) *Using Computers in Nursing*, Reston Publishing, Reston, VA.

Briggs, M. (1990) *Manage Your Business – Computerise Your Accounts*, Sigma Press, Wilmslow.

Burnard, P. (1991) Computing: an aid to studying nursing. *Nursing Standard*, **5**(17), 36–8.

Burnard, P. (1991) Working with computers. *Journal of District Nursing*, **10**(6), 18–19.

Burnard, P. (1992) The free form database program as a research tool. *Nurse Education Today*, **12**, 51–6.

Burnard, P. (1992) *Effective Communication Skills for Health Professionals*, Chapman & Hall, London.

Croucher, P. (1989) *Communications and Networks – A Handbook for the First Time User*, Sigma Press, Wilmslow.

Croucher, P. (1990) *Novell Networks Companion*, Sigma Press, Wilmslow.

De Presno, O. (1989) *The Shareware Handbook*, Sigma Press, Wilmslow.

Hannah, K., Guillemin, F. and Conklin, D.N. (1986) *Nursing Uses of Computers and Information Science*, North Holland, Amsterdam.

Jarrett, D. (1989) *The Comms Handbook*, Sigma Press, Wilmslow.

Jenkins, E. (1987) *Facilitating Self-Awareness: A Learning Package Combining Group Work with Computer Assisted Learning*, Open Software Library, Wigan.

Jordan-Marsh, M. and Chang, B.L. (1985) Assessing readiness for interaction with computers. *Medical Centres' Computers in Nursing*, **3**(6), 266–71.

Kelly, J. (1991) High-tech teach-in. *Nursing Times*, **48**, 59–60.

Koch, W. and Rankin, J. (eds) (1987) *Computers and Their Applications in Nursing*, Harper and Row, London.

Mcalindon, M.N. and Silver C.M. (1986) Computer software for nursing – the advantages of a hospital–university liaison. *Computers in Nursing*, **4**(1), 17–26.

McCormac, K. and Jones, B. (1992) A lesson in reality. *Nursing Times*, **88**(14), 55–7.

Procter, P. (1988) *Framework for Computer-Assisted Learning Implementation for Nursing, Midwifery and Health Visiting in England*, Aspects of Educational Technology XXI, Kogan Page, London.

Sinclair, V.G. (1985) The computer as partner in health care instruction. *Computers in Nursing*, **3**(5), 212–16.

Sweeney, M.A. (1985) *The Nurses Guide to Computers*, Macmillan, New York.

van Bemmel, J.H. (1987) Computer assisted care in nursing – computers at the bedside. *Computers in Nursing*, **5**(4), 232–5.

Vedera, S. (1989) *Applied Expert Systems*, Sigma Press, Wilmslow.

Index

Entries in *italics* are software or DOS applications; entries in **bold** are journals, magazines or databases.

Accessories 59
Accounts 10, 101
Active Life 211
Add-ons 37
Administration 14
Aidsline 108
Aims of research
    projects 163
Alternative therapies 2
Ami Pro 197
Ample Notice 210
Amstrad PCW 43
An Ounce of Prevention 226
Anti-virus programs 219
Aporia 221
Applause 122
Arcmaster 226
Arithmetic 114
Articles, writing 155
Artline 207
Arts and Letters 206
ASCII datasets 166
Association of Shareware
    Professionals 135
Auto back-up facilities 81
AUTOEXEC.BAT file 68
Automenu 228

B-Edit 225
B-Pop 225
B-Ware 226
Baby Watch 226
Back up 179
Backing up 11, 70
BASIC 179
Batch File Tutorial 214
Batteries 32
Battery Watch Pro 34
Beatty, G.J. 137
Benchmark 180
Bernoulli drive 180
Better Working Word 193
Bibliographic references 10
Big-WP 225
Binary 180
Biological Abstracts 108
BIOS 180
Bit 180
Books, writing 155
Boot 180
British Medical Journal
    108
BubbleJet 180
Burnard, P. 161
Bus 180
Business Cards 211
Buying computers 40, 43
Buying through the post 46
Buying software 128
Byte 180

C programming
    language 180
C-Stat 168
Cache (disk) 180
Camera ready copy 144
Cardbox 200
Caring 11
CD-ROM 12, 38
Central processing unit 18
Centring text 83
Centronics 181
Charisma 206
Chip 181
Chiwrit 222
City Desk 216
Client and Note File 210
Cliqword 194
Clone 181
Code to Code 217
Collective writing 86
*Colour Paint Graphics
    Package* 225
Colour palettes 181
Colours 91
*Command Post and
    Browser* 220
Comms 181
Compact Library: AIDS 108
Components of a PC 17
Computer Tutor 213

Computer Buyer 19
Computer magazines 19
Computer Glossary 213
Computers, types of 8, 17
Computing Crime Unit 72
CONFIG.SYS file 68
Configuration 58
Consumables 50
Content analysis 167
Continuous paper 39
Controller 181
Copy protection 29
Corel Draw! 206
Cost 47
Cost–benefit analysis 114
Counsellors 2
Cox, J. 75
CPU (central processing unit) 18, 181
Crash 181
Cricket Graph 206
Cricket Presents 206
Cumulative Index to Nursing and Allied Health Literature 108
Curriculum development 10
Cursor 27
Customizing 58
CVs 164

Daisywheel 182
Data analysis 167
Data collection in research 164
Data files 22
Data Protection Act 100
Databases 7, 95
DataEase 200
DataPerfect 103, 201
Davrelle 207
dBase 201
dBFast 203
Decision Analysis System 210
Default 182
Defragmentation 86
Deleting text 77

Delta 5 201
Demon 201
Dental Number 1 212
Designworks 206
Deskpress 204
Desktop computers 29
Desktop publishing 125
Desqview 55, 61
Dictionaries 15
Digitizer pad 182
Dingbat 183
Dirback 227
Direct Access 55
Directories 34
Directory Maintenance 229
Disk Efficiency 227
Disk drives, hard 22
Disk Consultant 214
Disk drives, floppy 24
Displaywrite 194
Doctors 2
Documentation standards 135
DOS 17, 18, 53, 54, 123
DOS shells 54
Dos Summary 213
Dosamatic Task-switching 230
Dosmenu 231
Dot matrix printers 38
Dot matrix 183
DR DOS 183
DR-DOS 55
DrawPerfect 123, 205
Drive 183
Drug Interaction Program 217
DTP (desktop publishing) 125, 183

E mail 36, 183
Easel 220
Easy Access 229
Easy Project 211
Easy-Base 214
Edraw 225
EMS 183
Equations editors 83

Ethical considerations in research 164
Excel 199
Expanded/extended memory 21, 183
Expansion card 184
Expansion slot 184
Export facilities 82
Express Calc 218
Extended memory 21
EZ Menu 231
EZ-Spreadsheet 218
EZ-Write 222

Fastfile 215
Faxes 36
Field 184
Fields, database 96
File Express 215
File 184
File manager 82
File-Commando 230
File-Check 219
Files, managing 65
Files, naming 64
Financial considerations in research 164
Finding a computer dealer 45
Finesse 205
Flexibak Plus 226
Floppy disk drives 24
Flower Remedy Finder 217
Fonts 92
Fonts, examples of 150
Footnotes 81
Format 184
Format-PC 104
Formbase 203
Forms, database 95
FoxBase+ 201
Foxgraph 205
FoxPro 201
Fragmentation, disk 73
Freebase 215
Freefile 215

Index

Free form databases 96
Freelance Graphics 206

Galaxy 221
Galaxy Pro-Lite 194
Gardner, D.C. 137
GEM Desktop Publisher 205
General accounting 114
Get It 214
Good writing, principles of 139
Grammar checking 82
Grammatik 159
Graphical Menu System 231
Graphics 7, 120, 184
Graphics editors 82

H-Key 223
Handouts 10
Hard disk 185
Hard Disk Diagnostics 228
Hard disk drives 22
Hard disk maintenance 80
Hard Disk menu 229
Hardware 1, 58, 185
Harvard Draw 207
Harvard Graphics 206
Harvard Graphics for Windows 207
Hdtest 5.35 and Diredit 228
Headers and footers 92
Health care databases 107
Health care settings, using computers in 78
Health data 101
Health Risk Appraisal 217
Healthcare Product Comparison System 108
Help-Dos 213
Hexadecimal 185
Hi-Res Rainbow 224
Hicks, C. 75
High street shops 41
History of shareware 134
Hollywood 207
Housekeeping 63

Howard, W. 40
Hyper-Dos 213

IBM compatibility 40
Icon-Maker 224
Import facilities 82
In Control 209
Index Card Filer 214
Info Select 106
Information Please 215
Ink-jet 185
Ink-jet printers 38
Installation 58
Interface 185
Interleave factor 185
Interview transcripts 167
1st Word Plus 198

Jetsetter 204
Jobs 229
Justification 92
Justifying margins 85
JustWrite 197

K-Data 203
K-Spread 200
K-Word 2 198
Kervan, P. 75
Keyboard layout 92
Keyboards 26

Lancet 108
Language 186
LapLink 33
Laptops 30
Laser printers 38, 186
Leasing 48
Lecture notes 10
Lecturers 2
Leonardo 224
Letter writing 10
LetterPerfect 90, 194
LEX Elite 194
Life Sciences Collection 11
LIM EMS 186
Line spacing 92

Locoscript PC 194
Lotus Write 197

Machine code 186
Macros 83, 186
Magic II 201
Mail merging 84, 186
Managing People 211
Manuals, computer 2
Manuscript 194
Margin sizes 77
Margins
  bottom 93
  top 93
  wide 15
Martindale: The Extra Pharmacopoeia 108
Maths coprocessor 186
Med Number 1 212
Medline 109
Memory cache 186
Memory, computer 19, 186
Menu Master 231
Memory Mate 104, 172
Micromedex 109
Mind Reader 221
Mini Db 214
Modems 35, 187
Monitor, computer 28
Mouse 28
Mouse support 84
Moving text 77
MS-DOS Anti Virus 219
MS-DOS 55
Multimedia 187
Multiple screens 83
Multitasking 187
Multiword 195

Nelson, K.Y. 51
Networks 9, 187
New York Word 223
Non-Medical Pain Relief 217
Norton Utilities 73
Notebook computers 31
Nurses 2

Oberline, S. 75
Occupational therapists 2
Offload 227
Omnis 7 203
Operating systems 53, 187
Optical disk 187
Optiks 223
Oracle Database 6 201
OS/2 187
Outlining 84
Oxford Textbook of Medicine 108, 110
Oxford Writer's Shelf 155

PA Menu Manager 231
Page layout 84
Page numbering 92
Page size 93
PageMaker 204
PagePlus 127
Paint Shop 220
Palmtop computers 35
Paper 93
Papers, writing 155
Paradox 101, 202
Paragraph layout 145
Pascal 188
Pasting text 80
Patient/client records 10
Payrolls 101
PC Answers 19
PC Desk Team 230
PC Direct 19
PC Magazine 19
PC Picture Graphics 224
PC Plus 19
PC Scribe 195
PC-Calç Plus 218
PC-File (ButtonWare) 216
PC-File (OpenSoft) 202
PC-Label Maker 210
PC-Mag Benchmark 227
PC-Outline 223
PC-Type 4 222
PC-Write 222
PCW (Amstrad) 43
Peckitt, R. 130

Pen plotter 188
Pensions 101
Peripheral 188
Personal Appointment Locat 210
Personal Calendar 210
Personal computers, types of 17
Personal RBase 202
Pfaffenberger, B. 15
Physiotherapists 2
Pixel 188
PK Ware 226
Planning database programs 73
PlanPerfect 118, 199
Plotter 188
Pop Form 211
Postal buying 46
PostScript 188
Power Menu 229
Powermenu 55
PowerPoint 207
Prescription Assistant 217
Prescription writing 10
Printer drivers 83
Printers 38
Processor 18
Procube 3D 199
Professional Write 197
Profile 216
Programming standards 135
Progress 4GL/RDBMS 202
Pronto Graph 223
Proqube Lite 218
Protext 195
PsycLit 110
Publisher 204

QEMM 20
Qualitative analysis 171
Quattro 119
Quattro Pro 199
Quattro Pro SE 199
Quickplan 218

RAM (random access memory) 20
Range Text Manager 195
Rationale, research 163
RBase 3.1 202
Re-boot 189
Record 189
Reference Update 11
Renting 48
Report writing, research 174
Reports, writing 155
Research 10
Research methods 164
Research and personal computers 163
Resolution 189
Re-using disks 27
Right and left margins 93
Rimmer, S. 93
ROM 189
RS232 189
Rubicon Publisher 216

Samna Word 195
Scanner 189
Scientific Calculator 212
Scout-Em 230
Screen Designer 224
Screen Peace 220
Scribe 222
Search and replace 80
Seating and computing 32
Secondhand, buying computers 48
Sector 189
Sedbase 110
Sentences, 141
Serial port 189
Service agreements 47
Set-Up and System Utilities 227
Shareware 133
history 134
Sidekick 21
Sigel, C. 112
Sign Friends and Learn to Sign 225
SIM/SIMM 189

Index

Sitter 212
Slide Generator 224
SmartWare 199
SmartWare II 202
Socha, J. 75
Social services data 101
Social workers 2
Sociofile 110
Software 1
 buying 128
Sommer, B. and Sommer, R. 175
Speed 4
Spell checking 77, 80
Spreadsheets 7, 113
SS Choice 219
Stand-alone computers 9
Statistics 101, 210
Statistics packages 7, 168
Still River Shell 229
Stowaway 227
Students 2
Stupendos 229
Style 146
Styles features 83
Subdirectories 66
SuperBase 4 Windows 203
SuperCalc 199
SuperDB 202
Super Stor 23
Superstores, computer 46
Support standards 135
Survey 171
SVGA 190
Symbol Design 225
System Speed Test 228

Tab settings 93
Table editors 83
Tape streamer 190
Tassword PC 195
Teachers 2
Telephone sockets 36
Test Drive 227
Textor 195
Textor for Windows 197

The Day Care Manager 211
The Donor Network 212
The Statistician 212
The Volunteer Network 211
Thesaurus 82
Tie Database 209
Timetabling in research 164
Timeworks Publisher 205
Toner 190
Toolkit 190
Top and bottom margins 93
TopCopy Plus 2 195
TopCopy Professional 196
Total System Statistics 228
Track 190
Tracker ball 190
Tree Top 230
Treeview 230
Trimming programs 137
TSR 190
Tuning 58
Turbo Calc 218
Tutor.Com 213
Tutors 2
Typeface 190
TypePlus 127
Types of personal computers 17

Underlining 93
Unistat 169
User checklist 44
Uses of personal computers in the health professions 10
Utilities 59

Vaccine and Virus Detector 219
Varieties of wordprocessors 78
Ventura Publisher 204
VGA (video graphics array) 28, 191
Virus 191
Virus Detector 219
Viruses 71

Visual System Information 228
Volkswriter 196
Vuwriter 196

Warranty 47
What Personal Computer? 19
Winbatch 221
Windos 230
Window Base 203
Windows 40, 55, 57
Windows Clock 220
Windows Draw 207
Windows Post-It 220
Windows 19
Winedit 221
Wingz for Windows 200
Word 79, 196
Word counting 80
Word for Windows 197
Wordcheck Plus 196
Wordcraft 196
WordPerfect 79, 87
WordPerfect for Windows 198
WordPerfect Office 55
Wordprocessing 7, 77
Wordprocessors, varieties 78
Wordprocessing functions 79
Words and Figures 199
WordStar 79
WordStar for Windows 198
Write On 197
Writing papers 155
Writing with a computer 139
Writing skills, 139
Wsmooth 220
WYSIWYG (What You See Is What You Get) 57

X Tree Gold 55

Year Book 1990 Edition 110

Zephyr 215
Zoom features 81